Caring for the Healing Heart

There is no doubt in my mind that Norman Cousins made the correct decision in 1980, when he declined bypass surgery and proposed that we defer a final decision pending an opportunity to put into effect a disciplined program involving nutrition, exercise, and a lifestyle emphasizing reduced tension and stress. My job was to monitor that program week by week.

There has been no surgery. In fact, it was possible very early on to discontinue all medication. Most remarkably, recent tests show that the heart has made its own bypass around the occluded arteries and is receiving all the oxygen it needs.

David S. Cannom, M.D.
from the *Introduction*

Avon Books by
Norman Cousins

THE HEALING HEART

Avon Books are available at special quantity discounts for bulk purchases for sales promotions, premiums, fund raising or educational use. Special books, or book excerpts, can also be created to fit specific needs.

For details write or telephone the office of the Director of Special Markets, Avon Books, Dept. FP, 105 Madison Avenue, New York, New York 10016, 212-481-5653.

Caring for the Healing Heart

An Eating Plan for Recovery from Heart Attack

Eleanor Cousins

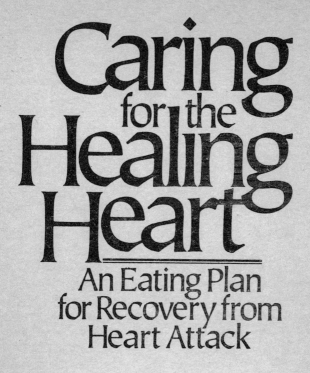

AVON BOOKS ◆ NEW YORK

AVON BOOKS
A division of
The Hearst Corporation
105 Madison Avenue
New York, New York 10016

Copyright © 1988 by Eleanor Cousins
Published by arrangement with W.W. Norton & Company, Inc.
Library of Congress Catalog Card Number: 87-28733
ISBN: 0-380-70744-6

First Avon Books Printing: October 1989

AVON TRADEMARK REG. U.S. PAT. OFF. AND IN OTHER COUNTRIES, MARCA REGISTRADA, HECHO EN U.S.A.

Printed in the U.S.A.

K-R 10 9 8 7 6 5 4 3 2 1

FOR NORMAN,
WHO INSPIRES AND MOTIVATES

Contents

Introduction

Hardly less remarkable than the advances in medical science's understanding of heart disease is the cardiologist's increasing respect for the role of the patient and family in any strategy for recovery.

One of the best examples of this new emphasis is the story told by Eleanor Cousins in her new book. She describes the profound contribution a person can make to the repair of a loved one's heart during the weeks and months following a myocardial infarction. Eleanor Cousins, let it be said at once, has no apologies to make for her total dedication to her family's well-being. Her principal satisfactions in life have come from her single-minded devotion to the care of her husband and four children. She recognizes that many factors are involved in this, nutrition high among them.

She is right in believing that the American people may be the best-fed in the world but are not the best-nourished. Even within the medical profession, one often hears the statement that the average supermarket shopping basket contains all the nutrients needed by the average family. But one has only to inspect the contents of the average supermarket shopping basket, with its processed foods, some of them heavily salted or sugared, to see the fallacy of this statement.

A primary value of this book, therefore, is that it provides a workable, reasonable guide to a daily diet—not just for people recovering from heart attacks or other serious illnesses, but for the entire family and, indeed, anyone who accepts the connection between sensible eating habits and good health. Eleanor Cousins recognizes, of course, that there need be no contradiction between nutritious food and tasty food. Nutrition fails in its essential purpose unless food is as gustatorily satisfying as it is healthy.

A heart attack is causally related to a number of factors, including a patient's genetic legacy, blood pressure, and cholesterol level. Other variables can accentuate these basic risk factors in a given patient. Among them are unusual emotional strains and stresses; excessive nicotine or alcohol or drug consumption; a greater burden of fats, sugar, salt, or chemicals in food than the body is equipped to handle; insufficient exercise or sleep; inadequate recreation or other satisfactions; etc. All these imbalances figure not just in heart attacks, but in most serious disease. Wise physicians, therefore, address themselves to basic causes and not just to symptoms. Eleanor Cousins takes the multiple causes of illness into account. In so doing, she serves as a valuable ally of the cardiologist, who may not be in a position to monitor all the everyday things that are essential for people recovering from heart attacks. She knows that profound reassurance to the stricken patient is no less vital than mouth-to-mouth resuscitation or any of the other physical procedures emphasized in public-education campaigns.

Panic is the prime enemy of anyone who is suddenly hit with devastating chest pains. It can constrict the blood vessels, forcing a damaged heart to work harder than usual to push the blood through suddenly narrowed passages. The fact of imminent death is a real and terrifying possibility to the person affected. How nearby persons react to someone who is stricken can increase or decrease the environment of panic and thereby have an effect on the outcome. If an onlooker starts to scream, the reality of panic becomes that much more dramatic.

Eleanor Cousins understands the psychological and emotional components involved in dealing with emergency health situations no less than she does the nutritional and other requirements of patient care. She makes valuable suggestions for creating a complete environment conducive to recovery.

I understand that one of the titles originally suggested for this book was *The Care and Feeding of a Husband.* Compelling as that title was, it was rejected because it might have detracted from the book's value for both sexes and for all those who wish to maintain good health. Yet the aptness of that title is undeniable. I had a chance to observe firsthand, during the months following Norman Cousins's serious heart attack, the extent to which Eleanor Cousins nursed and guided him back to full health. Now that the heart attack is completely behind him—it has been seven years at this writing since he suffered a major myocardial infarction—it is possible to identify and analyze all the elements involved in what has been a truly remarkable recovery. A recent rigorous cardiac examination shows that new blood vessels have been created and, indeed, that his heart has been thoroughly reconditioned. He plays tennis singles against men half his age and can go at top speed on the court for two hours or more.

There is no doubt in my mind that he made the correct decision in 1980, when he declined bypass surgery. But he hadn't rejected the surgery outright. He proposed that we defer a final decision on surgery pending an opportunity to put into effect a disciplined program involving nutrition, exercise, and a life style emphasizing reduced tension and stress along with a corresponding increase in reading, writing, music, and sports. My job was to monitor that program week by week. If the progress were significant and consistent, we would stay with it and see how far it would take us; if the progress were insufficient or too slow, we still had the option of surgery.

There has been no surgery. In fact, it was possible very early on to discontinue all medication. Most remarkably, recent tests show that the heart has made its own bypass around the occluded arteries and is receiving all the oxygen it needs.

When Norman Cousins wrote in *The Healing Heart* that his wife was the chief factor in that recovery, he was stating a literal truth. The story behind that recovery, as Eleanor Cousins tells it, can be of inestimable help to others.

David S. Cannom, M.D.

PART 1

Walking the Track

After Norman had recovered from his heart attack, a friend told me that she felt a great deal of sympathy for me. "It must have been a difficult time for you," she said. "You must have suffered."

"It may sound strange," I told her, "but that was one of the most joyous times in our life together."

Norman and I worked as a team on his recovery. On the very day he got out of the hospital, we embarked on a walking program. I accompanied my husband every day, twice a day, to the exercise track near our home. As we walked, we talked and played word games. We were able to have sustained conversations for the first time in our forty-plus years of marriage. Norman has always led a busy life. So it was a real treat for us to be together so much. We talked about our children, our *Saturday Review* years, the work at UCLA, our plans for the future. We found new friends among the people who came daily to the track. The time flew by, and the miles passed quickly under our feet. I enjoyed it as much as he did, and I'm sure the exercise did me no harm.

Norman has always loved photography, and soon

we brought his camera with us to the track and he began to take pictures of the flowers and trees in the park. Having moved so recently to Los Angeles from Connecticut, we were still dazzled by the year-long display of blossoms in southern California. Norman is an accomplished photographer. He would take a picture of a palm tree in the morning light and take another picture of the same palm tree in the afternoon and marvel at the difference. I have never seen him so observant of everything around him, now that he had time to enjoy life to the full.

When we returned home from the walking track, he would work at his typewriter. He began to write a play. His work with the Brain Research Institute at UCLA and his great interest in the biochemistry of the emotions aroused his curiosity about hypnotism and how Dr. Franz Anton Mesmer, in 1784 at his clinic in Paris, France, used what he called "animal magnetism" to treat illness through the power of suggestion. Every night Norman would sit at the typewriter writing his play. As he points out in his book *The Healing Heart*, few things are more conducive to longevity than creativity.

For my part, I was able to give Norman the kind of food that would rebuild his heart. I had studied nutrition for thirty years and looked forward to putting that knowledge to work.

I had read about the simple diets of certain peoples in the less industrialized areas of the world who were able to maintain good health without suffering from the degenerative diseases so common in highly industrialized societies. Some groups ate a predominantly vegetarian diet, and others ate mostly meat or fish or dairy foods. But what all those diets had in common

was that the food was natural, fresh, whole, uncon-
taminated by chemicals, and unprocessed.

I, therefore, decided on a broad diet that included
a large proportion of raw and cooked vegetables and
fruits, beans, peas, and grains; eggs, butter, milk,
and yogurt; and small portions of lean meats, chicken,
or fish. I made an effort to buy the highest-quality
food containing as few chemicals as possible and
shunned all processed and manufactured foods. I was
able to purchase a good supply of fresh vegetables
and fruits year round, many of which were organically grown.

At first, Norman could walk only a few yards at a
time. I left it entirely to his judgment. When he said
he needed a rest, we rested. When he felt strong
enough to continue walking, we walked. I have never
known anyone who is so well in tune to what is happening to his body. He knows exactly what his limi-
tations are. During the first month, it usually took
three slow circuits of the track to start his heart and
lungs functioning properly. But, as the weeks passed,
we could see a gradual improvement. Day by day we
increased speed and distance until we were walking
three brisk miles in the morning and three in the afternoon.

During those months, we had little or no social
life. We concentrated on the walking. Our schedule
was a simple one. We got up at seven, had breakfast,
were on the track before nine, and would walk for
about an hour. When we returned home, Norman
would have an apple or a glass of freshly made apple
juice because I had read that pectin helps to bring
down the cholesterol level in the blood. Pectin is a
carbohydrate that is also beneficial to the intestines.
Bottled pectin should be avoided because it contains

preservatives. Fresh green apples such as pippins or Granny Smiths are the best source. (Through my reading of books on nutrition over the years, I have learned that some of the richest sources of pectin are the pulp of citrus fruits, the whit of orange rind, the inside pulp of sweet red peppers, carrots, and green apples. I put that information to good use some years ago when I was making quince jelly. I found that quince by themselves would not jell, but if I added a few green apples to the quince, it would jell immediately.)

Norman would work at the typewriter or read or rest until lunch, and at three o'clock we would go again to the jogging track. At four, I would give him another glass of fresh fruit juice or carrot juice. I found myself concentrating on him to such an extent that I began to feel almost as if we were one person.

To demonstrate: Dr. Omar Fareed, our family doctor, had asked Norman to come to his office before breakfast one morning for a blood test. We got up early, and I told a friend who was visiting us that we would be back for breakfast very soon because, I said, "I'm very hungry."

"Well, *you* can eat," she pointed out. "*Your* blood isn't being tested."

With a jolt, I realized that what *I* ate had no effect on Norman. Our joint effort had, at least in my mind, fused us into a single entity.

A week after Norman had returned home from the hospital and we were well into our regimen of good nutrition and exercise, Dr. Kenneth Shine, Norman's cardiologist, came to the house to recommend that Norman have an angiogram to determine whether he should have bypass surgery. The doctor not only felt that Norman's chances of surviving the first year without a bypass were not good enough, but felt a personal responsibility to improve those chances.

We were touched by his concern and grateful. But Norman believed that he should give his body an opportunity to create its own bypass. He was beginning to feel stronger, and we could see a marked increase in his stamina on the track. The improvement was slow but steady, and it held.

"I can't imagine any reputable doctor not agreeing with me," the doctor said, "but will you do me the favor at least of getting a second opinion?" Norman agreed.

As Norman has described in *The Healing Heart*, he did some telephoning and learned that David Cannom, a cardiologist with an excellent reputation, had recently come from Yale to the area and was connected to the UCLA's auxiliary at San Pedro. Norman told Dr. Cannom that he was not rejecting the angiogram-bypass route altogether but felt we ought to see whether significant progress could be made without it. Then, if Dr. Cannom was dissatisfied with his condition, we still had the option of surgery.

Dr. Cannom concurred with this approach. He recommended, however, that we attempt to bring down Norman's cholesterol count; at that point, it was 285—about 80 points higher than it ought to be. In my reading, I had run across a number of suggestions as to how to do this nutritionally. As I mentioned earlier, the pectin in green apples was helpful. Also, Norman drank at least four to six glasses of water a day. I remembered reading that onion and garlic were good for reducing blood cholesterol and inhibiting clotting, so I added them to the cabbage salad that I serve as a first course every evening at dinner. A high-fiber diet was an important part of our regimen. I also gave him small daily doses of niacin, again with Dr. Cannom's approval.

Six weeks later, when Norman went back to Dr. Cannom's office for another checkup, his cholesterol count had dropped to 190. Dr. Cannom was impressed. He said he had rarely seen such a remarkable reduction in that period of time, even by means of medication.

We began to take a blood-pressure measuring device with us to the track and would measure Norman's blood pressure before and after exercise. I will never forget our excitement the first time the device showed a normal blood-pressure response to the walking. We knew then, without any doubt, that his body was making its own bypass and that he was going to make it all the way. It was a glorious moment.

Our first expedition away from home (other than to the walking track) was to the Los Angeles Zoo. We enjoyed looking at the people as well as the animals. Norman's camera was never busier.

About five months after his heart attack, Norman began to lecture again in the Los Angeles area. At first, he limited himself to a 45-minute talk with a short question period. I would do the driving to and from the lecture hall so that he might save his energy for the talk, and I always made sure that there was a microphone and a pitcher of drinking water at the podium.

Since there is nothing Norman enjoys more than physical exercise—especially if it involves hitting a golf ball, a tennis ball, or a baseball—it was not long before he wanted to get back into action, using a golf cart at first. I am not a golfer, but I often accompany Norman around the course. All his life he has been active in athletics and, while a young reporter in New

York City, played in the Metropolitan Newspaper Baseball League.

As Norman became more active, one of his doctors asked him how he had handled the depression that usually follows a heart attack. Norman had had no depression; he was probably too busy enjoying himself—the walking, his photography and playwriting, plus the excitement of seeing a steady improvement in his health and strength. Even I was amazed when, less than three months after his heart attack, he began playing tennis again.

I think Norman is stronger today than he has been for years. At the time of this writing, he celebrated his seventy-second birthday. He maintains a twelve-hour workday. On weekends, he plays a hard game of tennis—singles and doubles—and not infrequently beats men half his age. Sometimes he plays golf in the morning and tennis in the afternoon of the same day—without strain. He doesn't travel around the country as much as he used to, but that still leaves him with about 40,000 lecture miles a year. He considers a seat on an uncrowded plane one of the best places to write and think. He likes the work he is doing at UCLA and is enjoying life now more than ever before.

In *The Healing Heart,* Norman wrote about this regimen of good nutrition, controlled exercise, and freedom from stress. In this book, I will explain how I was able to assist him in his program so that others who find themselves in a similar situation can play a vital role in the recovery of their loved one. True, the effort required is not small. But the rewards are substantial.

Optimism Is Contagious

The day before Norman had his heart attack, we were forewarned. We had just started playing tennis doubles with his sister and her husband when Norman said he didn't feel well and had to sit down. He was perspiring heavily but felt no pain, and, after a few minutes of rest, he felt like continuing the game. But we stopped playing, went home, and thought little more about it.

The following day, while we were eating lunch, he again began to perspire heavily and felt a tightness in his chest. He was nauseated and very uncomfortable. I think he knew immediately that he was having a heart attack. He asked me to get the small emergency oxygen tank we keep in the house for the same reason we keep a fire extinguisher nearby. He also asked for some towels and dry clothing. Despite his awareness that he was in danger, I could see he was not panicky, but in total control.

As soon as he had gotten into bed, he asked me to call Dr. Sherman Mellinkoff, dean of the UCLA Medical School. Dr. Mellinkoff told me not to worry, but felt that prudence dictated that Norman be brought to the hospital. He said he would send an ambulance immediately.

I went back to the bedroom, reported to Norman, who was sitting up in bed using the small oxygen tank. He smiled at me and told me not to worry. I was amazed. I had heard him tell lecture audiences and his medical students that the most important thing to remember during a heart attack is not to panic because panic constricts the blood vessels and makes it more difficult for the body to handle the attack. And here he was, putting his theories into practice.

In a few minutes, we could hear the ambulance coming up the hill. I opened the front door, and the paramedics rushed in. They wanted to give Norman morphine and lidocaine, but he refused both; his pain, such as it was, required no such drastic medication. Of course, he made no objection to the oxygen or the cardiograph. "Don't worry," he reassured the paramedics, "I'm going to be all right."

They connected him to the oxygen tank and prepared to carry him out to the ambulance. As they were going out the door, I heard Norman say, "I don't think we'll need the siren." Then he turned to me and suggested that I follow in my car. The ambulance went swiftly and quietly to the hospital, and I followed. Norman tells me he waved to me during the trip to the hospital. I wasn't able to see that, but I believe him.

As I found out, a heart attack can happen at any time. Not infrequently, the attack comes as a complete surprise and shock to victim and family.

One can hardly blame a life partner of a heart-attack victim for feeling desperate in such a dangerous situation. It is important, however, to be aware of the effect your behavior will have on your loved one. Nothing is more essential in a health emergency than to prevent panic. Panic is destructive and can interfere with essential treatment. If you have ever had ambitions to perform on the stage, this is the time to play your best role. Don't minimize the seriousness of what is happening, but don't underestimate the need to be reassuring and calm. Try to create an atmosphere of confidence. If you can't reach your doctor, tell the telephone operator you have an emergency situation and ask her or him to help you get an ambulance. Make the patient as comfortable as possible. Try to see that everyone else in the house remains calm. If someone screams or flails about, remove that person from the patient's presence. It has been scientifically proved that a heart-attack patient who is relatively free of panic has a much better chance of survival than one whose heart has to work harder because of the narrowed blood vessels that result from extreme fright. Also, the hormonal surges that accompany panic put the heart at greater risk.

When the ambulance arrives, reassure the patient again, reminding him or her that he or she is on the way to a hospital that handles such cases every day. If possible, ride in the ambulance with the patient and hold his or her hand. Smile and make small talk with the paramedics. Your optimism can be contagious. Don't allow yourself the luxury of tears.

Any person who is ill needs to believe that he or she will recover. The positive attitude of a patient plays a significant role in treatment and return to health. Physicians have always believed that a strong will to live increases a patient's chances of combating serious illness. Few things are more important in the care of the seriously ill than their mental state and the general environment of their treatment.

When your friends get word of what has happened, they will want to visit the patient in the hospital. It's important, then, for you to stay in charge. Gently remind all visitors that you want to maintain a pleasant atmosphere in the hospital room. Suggest that they keep the conversation upbeat. Keep an eye on the patient. If you see that the patient is tired and wants to nap, shorten the length of the visit.

My husband's doctor allowed me to bring a thermos of freshly squeezed orange juice to the hospital every day. I also brought homemade bread and freshly made vegetable soup. It is important for the patient to eat enough to sustain good health and strength. And favorite foods brought from home can provide a link to the world outside the hospital.

During Norman's hospital stay, I wanted to be there all the time. This, of course, was not permitted. But when I did come into his room, I tried to leave all personal and household problems behind: I did not talk to him about the plumbing or about family finances. I made an effort to be cheerful, smiling, and confident. I let him lead the conversation. If he didn't feel like talking, we didn't talk. I was happy just to sit there for an hour or so and work on a crossword puzzle or read a book. He knew I was there, ready to do anything he wanted me to do.

I never had any doubts that Norman would recover completely. While he was still in the hospital, I went to the UCLA Student Store and bought four new sport shirts for him and brought them to his room for his approval. Norman's doctor apparently thought I didn't understand the seriousness of the situation because he asked me to come to his office for a talk. After sitting me down, he sternly told me that he hadn't wanted to frighten me but felt it was important for me to know that Norman had suffered a massive heart attack, that he was not out of the woods yet, that he had a long way to go, and that he probably would need a bypass operation. He said he could see that all I could think about was getting Norman home. He was right. I felt that nutritious food, regular exercise, and a cheerful environment were all that Norman needed.

Depression is almost universal following a heart attack. The reason is obvious. The heart is the principal organ of the body, and it is likely that the heart-attack victim may have the feeling that he or she will never physically be the same again. It is important to convince the patient that this need not be true. There is nothing stronger than the regenerative powers of the body, given a healthy diet, regular exercise, and an optimistic attitude.

Don't allow your loved ones to think of themselves as invalids. As a safeguard against depression, encourage them to return to creative activities put aside or to find new ones. You know what their capabilities and interests are. Once your loved ones are involved creatively, and if they eat nutritious food and exercise regularly, they will get stronger every day. The improvement will be slow but steady. At first, they may not be aware of the healing force, but you will be able to see it happening. And soon they will, too.

The Importance of Fiber

When I became interested in nutrition, I read everything I could find on the subject. My bedside table was stacked high with books and magazines. The more I read, the more enthusiastic I became. The whole family—my sisters and brothers, Norman's sisters and brother, their wives and husbands, even Norman's mother—thought I had gone off the deep end.

I swept the house clean of white flour and sugar. Out went the chocolate cookies, Good Humor ice cream, corn flakes. Of course, the children and Norman resisted my efforts to make them healthy. Now I know I should have done it quietly and unobtrusively. But at that time, I could think of little else. I began to bake whole-wheat bread and to make yogurt. And I had a great desire to spread the good word.

Whenever Norman and I were invited out to dinner, I considered myself fortunate if I could steer the conversation with my dinner partner toward my nutritional interests. Across the table, Norman would squirm as he overhead snatches of our conversation. He was worried that I was imposing on our hosts by taking advantage of a captive audience (which, of

15

course, I was). Many times, as we were about to enter the dining room, Norman would pull me aside and whisper urgently in my ear, "Please, don't talk about nutrition tonight."

"Okay, I won't," I would say blithely. But with the slightest encouragement from my dinner partner, my promise would be forgotten.

Despite their protests, Norman and the children benefited from my commitment to nutritious foods. An early result of the improved diet was that Norman's hay fever became less severe. In the first year of our marriage, during the heavy pollen months, he would be up all night, sneezing and gasping for breath. He no longer has that problem.

Once in a while, Norman would reach over and up into my stack of books. I was not surprised. He has a great curiosity and an open mind. Perhaps he learned more from my books than he realized.

He also has a very deep interest in medicine. Even as a boy, he found medical books fascinating. When he was twelve years old, he learned of a national essay contest for high-school students, sponsored by the Women's Christian Temperance Union, on "The Evils of Drinking Alcohol." He went to the library, did research on the effects of alcohol on the human body, wrote his essay, and won the national first prize—twenty-five dollars. He claims that this experience shaped his life in two ways: he renounced liquor without a struggle, and he realized that he could earn money by writing. This led to his working his way through college by editing a plumbing magazine (of all things) and by free-lance sports reporting for the local newspapers. After his graduation from Columbia's Teachers' College, he worked full time as an education writer for the *New York Post* and was also sent out on medical assignments.

In 1964, when Norman became seriously ill, he was able to investigate his own case, as he describes in his book *Anatomy of an Illness*. Norman and his physician, Dr. William M. Hitzig, had been friends for more than thirty years. Bill Hitzig would often take Norman with him on his hospital rounds and house calls, and would discuss in great detail the underlying problems of each patient. Norman was able to ask the right questions of his doctor during his illness, and he knew which medical journals and text books to consult. Bill welcomed these questions, for, as he told his colleagues, they sharpened his own perceptions and allowed him to work with Norman as a partner in a joint effort. In addition, I was very happy when Norman was able to tell Bill that Vitamin C might combat the mysterious infection that was causing Norman's illness. I felt sure that this information came from my stack of nutrition books.

While Norman was in the hospital, several of our four daughters were still at home in New Canaan, Connecticut. Every night after I had served dinner to the girls, I would fill a basket with fresh vegetables from my garden and drive to the hospital in New York City. Norman loved to eat freshly picked carrots, tomatoes, cucumbers, and sweet red peppers—and so did Bill Hitzig. But, contrary to the TV movie that was based on *Anatomy of an Illness*, I did not walk from room to room in the hospital forcing carrots down the throats of other patients.

Actually, fresh vegetables have been a mainstay of our diet since the early days of our marriage. My mother had always grown her own vegetables, and I followed her example. When we lived in our first home in Old Greenwich, Connecticut, overlooking Long Island Sound, we dined at a card table set up in the middle of our small living room. I could hardly find enough room on the table for all the extra vegetables I had prepared for our evening meal; sometimes there were as many as nine, in addition to the meat course. I *was* overdoing it, but, in retrospect, more than forty years later, I am amazed that I had enough sense to know the importance of fresh vegetables and of choosing a widely varied diet.

A popular notion today of an adequate main meal is a tossed lettuce salad; a meat, fish, or chicken main dish with one cooked vegetable; something sweet for dessert. But this meal does not include enough fiber. With a little extra effort, the meal can be substantially improved. Add to the salad wedges of fennel, cabbage or celery, carrots, turnips, or other raw fibrous vegetable, or serve a thick vegetable soup. Add a side dish of split peas, lentils, or barley to provide variety (and fiber). My husband considers it a special treat when I include a side dish of red or white beans. They can be served warm with Mexican spices or cold with a vinaigrette. In addition, instead of one cooked vegetable, serve two: spinach, cauliflower, string beans, peas, zucchini, rutabaga, beets. And how about celery root or fava beans for a change? They both are flavorful and are easily prepared.

As for a dessert with fiber, I would suggest brown-rice and raisin pudding or stewed or fresh fruit.

The point here is that we can easily improve the quality of the main meal by serving an increased amount and variety of vegetables, fruits, grains, seeds, and legumes. Researchers have found that people who eat a high-fiber diet are better able to resist the degenerative diseases that plague highly industrialized societies.

Some people believe that all the nutrients you need can be had from the average American diet. Perhaps this was true for our grandparents, but not today. In the early 1900s, Americans did much more physical work, walked more, and ate a simpler diet. Today, the average American consumes many processed foods and rarely walks even as far as the grocery store. A glance into the average American's food shopping basket reveals a collection of frozen and canned ready-to-eat food, overrefined and laced with sugar, salt, preservatives, and artificial flavors and colors. The result of such a diet is reflected in the enormous annual medical costs we pay. Infants, teen-aged girls, pregnant women and breast-feeding mothers, and the elderly are the groups most affected.

A 1984 survey of Los Angeles and New York preteen-aged school children showed many with cholesterol levels of 175. This level is at least one-third higher than is consistent with arterial health. At this rate, such children may reach cholesterol levels in excess of 250 by the age of thirty-five. (The Framingham Study of the National Institutes of Health shows that a cholesterol level of 245 places people at high risk for heart attacks.) Many teen-aged and preteen-aged children today live on a diet of junk foods: hamburgers, French fries, pizza, soda, sugar-laden cereals, and the like. These are the kinds of food that clog the arteries and cause heart problems.

Some say that a commercial, "properly prepared" pizza meets the Dietary Goals of the Senate Select Committee on Nutrition and Human Needs in terms of its protein, fat, and carbohydrate content. That may be so, but if a pizza made with white flour represents a good part of a teenager's diet, he or she is eating quite a bit of a food that will make him or her fat but not healthy. In addition, I suspect that canned foods are generally used in the making of commercial pizzas. The only way you can make a pizza that is nutritious is to use only fresh, body-building ingredients.

Recently, more than half of the young men registering for the draft were rejected because they did not meet physical standards. One examining physician reported that their hair is turning gray at an early age, their teeth are decayed, and their faces are sallow and wrinkled. About one-third of the young men applying to the army are turned down as well as three-fourths applying to the navy, which has higher standards.

A wide spectrum of medical problems, ranging from heart ailments, diabetes, osteoporosis, and arthritis to mental disorders, may be caused by a low-fiber diet. How many people do you know who suffer from migraines, allergies, insomnia, fatigue, "nerves," persistent colds, constipation, or some other "minor" ailment?

A high-fiber diet may help to alleviate these and many other problems. If you have difficulty gaining weight, if minor cuts and bruises are slow to heal, if your skin is sallow, your hair dry and lifeless, your fingernails ridged and brittle, or if you suffer from hot or cold weather more than most or have little energy and your doctor tells you that you have a protein deficiency, don't attempt to correct this situation by eating more meat. Since meat contains more phosphorous than calcium, too much meat can cause a calcium imbalance. Calcium deficiency can lead to osteoporosis, tooth decay, arthritis, and periodontal disease. The safest and best way to restore nutritional balance is to increase the variety and amount of fresh raw and cooked vegetables and fruits in your diet. A small amount of protein is enhanced when combined with a larger amount of vegetables and is of far greater nutritional value than a large serving of protein with a smaller amount of vegetables.

Surprisingly, the same diet can also help you to lose weight. Cut down on the quantity of the food you eat, if you think that is necessary, but keep the proportions the same: small servings of protein with a larger variety and quantity of fresh vegetables, fruits, grains, seeds, and legumes.

In the first half of the twentieth century, nutritionists did not realize the importance of fiber in the diet. Textbooks on nutrition published at that time dismissed "roughage" in a few lines. Not until 1969 did a surgeon in the British Royal Navy, Dr. T. L. Cleave, write a book on the importance of fiber in the diet— *Diabetes, Coronary Thrombosis and the Saccharine Disease*.

Little attention was paid to Dr. Cleave's ideas until Dr. Denis Burkitt, a member of the Royal Society in Great Britain and a highly respected cancer researcher, had read Dr. Cleave's book. In 1970, Dr. Burkitt published a paper of his own. He pointed out that cancer of the large intestine, so prevalent in Europe and North America, rarely occurred among Africans whose traditional diets were rich in fiber. Dr. Burkitt suggested that a high-fiber diet might protect not only against cancer of the colon, but against many other degenerative diseases as well.

In 1971, Dr. Neil Painter, an Oxford surgeon, supported Burkitt's theories by pointing out that diverticular disease was associated with prolonged bowel transit time and increased pressure in the sigmoid colon. He suggested that changes in pressure resulted from a deficiency of fiber and recommended a high-fiber diet for those with diverticular disease. This was revolutionary. Up to that time, the orthodox treatment for people with diverticular disease had been a bland low-fiber diet.

Interest in dietary fiber has increased since that time, and the medical profession now accepts the need for fiber in the diet for all, including heart patients.

Sometime during the last century, a Dutch physician in Java noticed that many of his wealthy patients became ill with beriberi but that the prisoners in his care were unaffected. Surely, he thought, the rich, who are able to afford the best of everything, ought to prosper in every respect. He examined the diets of both groups. Rice is a basic food for all people in Java, but the doctor discovered that his rich patients ate only polished white rice, which was much more expensive than the unpolished brown rice given to the prison inmates. This observation led to the discovery of B vitamins, the first to be identified.

By eating polished rice, he rich people of Java deprived themselves of most of the protein, fiber, calcium, vitamin B_1, vitamin B_2, niacin, potassium, and iron found in unpolished rice. Since the rice germ was removed in the refining process, vitamin E was also absent in the polished white rice.

In the same way, when the bran and the germ of wheat berries are discarded in the making of white flour, 89 percent of the vitamin B_1 is lost, as is 58 percent of the vitamin B_2, 60 percent of the vitamin B_6, 69 percent of the pantothenic acid, 79 percent of the folic acid, 89 percent of the niacin, 100 percent of the vitamin E, 60 percent of the calcium, 76 percent of the iron, 85 percent of the magnesium, 71 percent of the phosphorous, 77 percent of the potassium, 78 percent of the sodium, 78 percent of the zinc, and 22 percent of the protein. There is also the loss of fiber and trace minerals so essential to good health.

It is possible, too, that the refining process removes more essential nutritional elements than science so far has identified. Out of more than fifty known nutrients, Recommended Daily Allowances (RDA) have been established by the government for only seventeen. Whole foods grown in mineral-rich soil provide a wide variety of vitamins, minerals, enzymes, and other essential nutritional elements, both known and unknown.

The Second Washington Symposium on Dietary Fiber was held in Washington, D.C., on April 24–29, 1987. The conference, sponsored by the George Washington University School of Medicine and Health Sciences, featured a round-table discussion of the role that fiber plays in various aspects of human pathophysiology. Dr. Denis Burkitt, guest of honor and main speaker, described how Nauru, a small island in the Pacific, became a natural laboratory, proving that fiber is essential to a healthful diet. The inhabitants became wealthy, with a higher per-capita income than Americans, because of the sale of the phosphates that cover the island. Now prosperous, the islanders abandoned their transitional diet of coconuts, yams, bananas, and other native foods, importing their food from New Zealand and Australia. They no longer needed to work to eat and became sedentary. Today, in their new life of leisure and processed foods, 35 percent of the island population over the age of fifteen has diabetes.

Almost twenty years ago, Dr. Burkitt reported that a low intake of dietary fiber causes detrimental physiological changes, but it is only in recent years that the medical profession has realized just how detrimental these changes are. We now know that a healthy diet must include about 40 grams of fiber daily to protect against heart and circulatory disorders.

Each of the foods below, in the amounts indicated, contains 10 grams of fiber:

    4 slices whole-wheat bread
    4 shredded-wheat biscuits
    2 ears sweet corn
    1 cup cooked oatmeal
    1 cup whole-grain cereal
    ½ cup mixed beans
    ½ cup cooked dried peas
    ½ cup lentils
    1 generous portion cabbage salad (see pp. 119–120)
    5 apples
    4 peaches
    3 pears
    10 dried figs
    4 large carrots
    3 bananas
    6 oranges
    1 cup peanuts

The recommendation of the American Diabetes Association—for at least 40 grams of fiber a day—demonstrates that what is good for those with diabetes is also good for those with heart problems or for anyone else who wants to be in the best of health.

Cholesterol: Good Quality/Poor Quality

Since Norman's affiliation with UCLA, a rich source of information about the latest research in nutrition is his mail. He receives bulletins from research centers and universities around the world, and I am fortunate to have access to the most up-to-date information.

It is unfortunate that not more people in the health fields are aware of this research. They would discover, for example, that soybean lecithin can reduce cholesterol levels. They might also be surprised to learn that egg yolk contains the finest quality of lecithin known to science.

In the January 1985 *Longevity Letter*, a monthly review of biomedical research related to life extension, a group of researchers at the Weizmann Institute of Science in Israel has developed a compound derived from egg yolks; they have named it Active Lipid (AL). This compound shows good potential in reversing certain adverse effects of aging.

As we grow older, the cells that make up our body alter, producing rigidity in cell membranes. One such change is the accumulation of cholesterol in the membranes of brain cells and lymphocytes, a change that seems to reduce membrane fluidity and cell function, and may contribute to the aging of the immune system and to the increasing susceptibility to disease.

In the above-mentioned Israeli study, ten elderly people were given 10 grams of AL every day for a three-week period. Before the AL treatment, the lymphocyte proliferative responses of these people were two to six times lower than those of young volunteers. (These proliferative responses decline with aging.) After the three weeks, eight of the ten elderly participants showed improvement in memory and mental alertness. The researchers claim that ALM treatment consistently lowered the amount of cholesterol in cell membranes, making them more like the fluid membranes that coat cells in younger people.

Further bolstering of this point of view comes from Dr. Richard J. Wurtman of the Department of Nutrition and Food Science at Massachusetts Institute of Technology. For the last decade, he has been studying the effect of choline and lecithin from egg yolk in the treatment of certain brain disorders. Wurtman's research indicates that the lecithin in egg yolk dissolves cholesterol in the brain and improves the brain's function.

In his book *Nutrition against Disease,* Dr. Roger Williams, nutritionist at the University of Texas, supports this idea and other suggestions made in this book. He says: "On the basis of present information, the best abbreviated advice for preventing heart disease is this: Concentrate on the quality of the food consumed. Wholesome foods like milk, eggs, fish and vegetables which are generously endowed with essential nutrients should take preference over those processed foods that crowd out the good foods, contribute mostly calories, and provide very little in the way of amino acids, minerals and vitamins. Anyone who deliberately avoids cholesterol by avoiding good foods may be inadvertently courting disaster.''

In the same book, Dr. Williams says: ''The prevalence of cholesterol in the arteries has given rise to the idea that cholesterol is perhaps the villain in hardening of the arteries. This apparently obvious clue is, in fact, misleading. Cholesterol is an absolute essential for our bodies all through life. . . . Good cholesterol in its proper place is good, not bad, but the deposit of bad cholesterol on the inside of artery walls is a source of trouble.''

On the other side of the egg controversy, the Harvard School of Public Health reported that a carefully controlled eighteen-month study showed that as egg yolk was added to the diets of men in a Boston mental hospital, blood cholesterol levels rose. And so the controversy rages on.

But, you may ask, what about the cholesterol in the egg yolk? Yes, egg yolk does contain cholesterol, but it is a very fine kind of cholesterol. As Dr. Williams has pointed out, the body needs good cholesterol; it is vital for normal cellular metabolism and for the production of a number of important substances. Four-fifths of the cholesterol in the body is made by some cells, by the liver, and in the small intestines; it is manufactured constantly since the need is so great. Cholesterol is a constituent of hormones and of the sheaths that protect nerve fibers. It is, therefore, important to provide the cells and the liver with high-quality materials for the making of good cholesterol.

Poor-quality materials such as saturated fats (lard, margarine, and refined vegetable oils) cause the body to produce poor-quality cholesterol, which clogs the arteries and causes heart problems. Starchy foods that have been cooked in hot oils or fats, such as French-fried potatoes, potato chips, doughnuts, pastries, and so forth, are the worst offenders. And the human body does not know how to deal with artificial foods such as margarine, coffee whiteners, processed cheeses, and the like. You can't expect your liver to make good cholesterol out of such shoddy materials.

Even though Norman has always been receptive to my ideas about nutrition and admits that he has learned a good deal from reading the books that I have collected over the years, we do have a few differences of opinion. He is far more conservative about eggs than I am. He also believes, largely on the basis of studies carried out at Framingham, Massachusets, by the National Institutes of Health, that a cholesterol level above 200 is hazardous and that, at 245, it may be a portal to a heart attack. At the time of his own heart attack in 1980, his cholesterol level was 285. Consequently, he leans over backward to avoid building up cholesterol in his arteries. He believes that one egg two or, at most, three times a week represents a sensible limit, considering his determination to keep his total cholesterol under 200.

I decided not to quarrel with him about this. If, for breakfast, he wants one egg three times a week and yogurt four times a week, that is fine with me. I also don't argue with him about the need to keep the arteries free of cholesterol. But I do not think that eggs represent a hazard in this regard. He cites the Framingham Study as his authority, and so do I.

The Framingham Study, begun in 1949, investigated the effect of every known environmental factor that might contribute to heart disease, including the amount of cholesterol consumed. A large group of people were asked to keep careful records of everything they ate.

A report on this study, which appeared in October 1982 in the *American Journal of Clinical Nutrition,* dealt with 912 men and women. No attempt was made to change the way or what they usually ate, including the number of eggs consumed. They were simply questioned by personnel skilled in nutrition. The results showed that most of the men who participated in the study usually ate six eggs a week. Most of the women ate fewer than four eggs a week. Some of the men ate no eggs. Some ate as many as twenty-four eggs a week. Some of the women ate no eggs. And some ate as many as nineteen eggs a week. No information was given on how the eggs were prepared.

Dr. Thomas R. Dawber, who has been associated with the Framingham Study since its inception and is one of the authors of this report, concluded, with his associates, that "differences in egg consumption were unrelated to blood cholesterol levels or to coronary heart disease incidence." Furthermore, Dr. Dawber went on to state, "although it has never been proved that lowering serum cholesterol levels will effectively decrease atherosclerotic disease, the authors of this study feel that dietary changes aimed at doing so would seem reasonable, in view of the importance of this risk factor, and that the patient must be concerned with his entire dietary intake—and with his health in general. Few physicians are sufficiently knowledgeable regarding the nutrient content of foods to prescribe diets that are low enough in both saturated fats and cholesterol to achieve an effective lowering of blood lipids. Even if they were capable of prescribing such diets, the difficulties of teaching patients and obtaining compliance with the diet are so great that few physicians can expect to achieve cholesterol lowering by dietary means alone. The result is the easy way out is taken and the patient is advised to 'change from butter to margarine' and 'to give up eggs.' "

But nutritionists have long known that the amino-acid pattern of eggs is so well proportioned that eggs are used as a reference point for judging the quality of protein in other foods. Eggs are high in methionine (an amino acid); vitamins A, D, and K, and the entire B complex; and the minerals iron, phosphorous, calcium, magnesium, copper, sulphur, as well as many other trace minerals.

As mentioned earlier, Dr. Roger Williams, nutritionist at the University of Texas, says that a diet consisting of eggs, some good fiber, and some vitamin C could serve as a complete healthy diet for humans.

If you are trying to devise a healthy diet for a person who has suffered a heart attack, consider the evidence offered by these and other professionals who point to a varied diet that includes eggs.

But, as with all other foods, *quality* is the key word. It is not always easy to obtain eggs of good quality. Most commercially produced eggs come from hens that are caged and treated like machines; are fed water and food laced with chemicals; and are deprived of fresh air, sunshine, and freedom of movement. Constantly keeping the lights on in the henhouse encourages the hens to lay around the clock. Yellow dyes are added to the feed to produce a yellower yolk. Is it possible that an egg laid by a hen treated in this way can be of high quality?

(In some areas of the United States the Humane Society is conducting a campaign against this exploitation and cruelty. If you are interested in learning more about this campaign and in obtaining eggs from range-free chickens, perhaps your local Humane Society can help you.)

When we lived in New Canaan, Connecticut, I had thirty-five hens and a rooster. The chickens were able to scratch in the soil in the sunshine. I fed them grains and greens and the scraps from the table, and they produced wonderful eggs. The yolks were dark yellow, almost orange; the whites of the eggs were heavy, not runny; and the shells were thick and strong. The eggs were fertile. (I know that some authorities dismiss the notion that fertile eggs are nutritionally superior to sterile eggs. Other authorities, however, contend that fertile eggs contain growth and reproductive hormones and steroids beneficial to nerves and glands. So far as I know, no definitive studies have been undertaken that can throw light on this subject.) My neighbors were always asking me if I could spare a dozen eggs; they said the eggs from my chickens were the sweetest they had ever tasted.

Caution: Whereas egg yolks can be eaten raw as well as cooked, egg whites should not. Raw egg whites contain avidin, an enzyme that interferes with the body's ability to utilize biotin, a B vitamin essential for the proper metabolizing of cholesterol. To use the whole egg in the raw state, such as for an eggnog, the egg should be soaked for five minutes in hot water (140° to 160°) to neutralize the avidin in the egg white.

There are other foods that cause the body to produce poor-quality cholesterol, which leads to clogging of the arteries and heart problems. The following are worst offenders.

(I) *"Cold-pressed"* oils. Most health-food stores sell "cold-pressed" vegetable oils. Do not be fooled by the term "cold-pressed." It does not mean that the oil was extracted from its source without heat and without chemicals. You will notice that the oil is uniform in color and has little or no odor or flavor. It is not easy to accomplish this feat. "Cold-pressed" vegetable oils are extracted with solvents, such as hexane, carbon tetrachloride, or gasoline. The extracted oil is then boiled to remove the solvent (some of which may be left behind) and whipped with lye and with caustic soda to remove unwanted color and flavor. Finally, the oil is filtered and heated again to 400° for twelve hours. Before bottling, a chemical preservative is added such as butylated hydroxyanisole (BHA), which can cause allergies and affect liver and kidney function, or butylated hydroxytoluene (BHT), which is even more toxic and has been banned in Great Britain. Since the refining process removes lecithin, vitamin E, copper, iron, calcium, magnesium, and phosphorous from the oil, it can no longer be called a natural whole food.

(2) *Margarine.* I am all too aware of the high-powered advertising that pushes margarine as a good food for heart patients, but I can find no substantiation for this. Margarines are manufactured from refined vegetable oil. Hydrogen is added to the oil in the presence of a metallic catalyst, usually nickel or cadmium. The hydrogen ions are bonded to the oil molecules, saturating the molecules and transforming the oil into a solid. Add artificial color, and now you have that plastic miracle, margarine.

Do not be taken in by the words on the package "100% corn oil," "Contains no cholesterol," "High in polyunsaturates," or "Highest in unsaturates." All margarine is made from refined oil that is not only hydrogenated, but is also saturated.

As long as fats and vegetable oils are in their natural state and are not consumed excessively, they will not cause arterial disease. Vegetable oils can promote health if the oil is extracted from its source mechanically or is expeller-pressed, without heat or chemicals. The most stable oils are sesame oil and olive oil. Be sure that the label on the bottle carries the words "unrefined" and "expeller-pressed."

The Danger of
Processed Foods

By now, you will have realized that I feel strongly about the superiority of natural over processed or precooked foods. Supermarkets offer hundreds of ready-to-eat concoctions but few people take the trouble to find out what is put into these products. We assume that the processors are attending to our nutritional needs, but our trust is not well placed. As the number and variety of precooked foods has grown, the nutritional quality of the average American diet has deteriorated.

Thousands of people are allergic to the fresheners and preservatives in processed foods, but numerous food products contain these chemicals and the consumer is not informed of this on the labels. The average American eats at least seven pounds of food additives a year. These chemicals are the glue that holds manufactured food together. Acidulants stabilize jelly, and antioxidants allow canned tomatoes to remain on the shelf for months without becoming rancid. Chemicals put the lemon in frozen lemon pie, enzymes bleach the flour in cake mixes, and stabilizers keep processed cheese firm for long periods.

If you have been relying on the government to protect you, you may be distressed to learn that many Food and Drug Administration standards are being set by food-industry personnel who are temporarily serving time at the FDA but who will eventually return to their jobs in the food industry, where their real loyalty may lie.

The food industry maintains that there is no conclusive evidence to indicate that some of these additives are harmful. Shouldn't that be turned around? Shouldn't the food industry be compelled to show without a doubt that a chemical is safe for consumers before being allowed to add it to a product?

Some food manufacturers use every loophole they can find to circumvent the law. Processed foods made and sold within state borders are not covered by federal law. Many food processors have lowered standards of quality and cleanliness in those plants where food is prepared for sale within state lines.

The intensely competitive food industry strives primarily for customer acceptance of new products on the basis of appearance, convenience, flavor, and texture. Concerns for public health have been subordinated in certain instances to concerns of the marketplace. And today's chemists can make stale foods appear fresh, mask inferior quality, and substitute worthless chemicals for more costly nutritious ingredients.

Beatrice Trim Hunter, in her book *The Great Nutrition Robbery,* describes how chemist Dr. O. A. Battista, who was attempting to perfect a stronger tire cord in a rayon and cellophane factory, happened to mix some microcrystalline cellulose (a by-product of the wood-pulp industry) with water in an electric blender and produced a thick gel. The chemist realized that the gel had possibilities as a nonnutritive bulking agent that could be used in food processing. Using the cellulose, he mixed a batch of cookies, baked them, tasted them, and pronounced them good.

Microcrystalline cellulose is a highly purified form of sawdust. The snow-white, free-flowing powder is odorless, tasteless, and noncaloric. It contributes gel stability, bulk, opacity, and texture to many convenience foods and makes possible the formation of many new and highly profitable low-calorie foods. It is used to replace more costly ingredients in salad dressings, puddings, soups, and desserts, and it can substitute for a number of ingredients in candies, pretzels, and other snack items without changing the flavor. It can be added to fish cakes, cottage cheese, and stuffings for meat, fish, and fowl. It is used for part of the flour in baked goods and for part of the potatoes in mashed potatoes intended for low-calorie diets. Bread containing the sawdust (called ''alpha cellulose'' in the list of ingredients) is advertised as having 400 percent more fiber than whole-wheat bread and commands a higher price than other loaves.

The most effective way of avoiding cellulose and other useless or dangerous additives is to stay away from processed foods. Keep to the natural as the best route to health.

Whole Milk Is Best

Natural is best when it comes to milk, too. When I was a child in Utah, my mother had a Jersey cow named Martha that she cared for and milked herself. Martha produced enough milk for six children in our family and for some of our neighbors as well. We drank the milk as it came—unpasteurized. My mother made cheese, and we all took turns churning butter by hand.

When I had children of my own, I wanted a cow, too. Norman didn't share my enthusiasm. He admitted that he didn't know very much about cows, but he did know they had to be milked twice a day and he could imagine what the telephone conversation would be like if he called me in New Canaan to remind me of a dinner date in New York. He knew something about my priorities.

Some years later, when we were in the Soviet Union for a Dartmouth Conference meeting, we became friendly with playwright Alexandre Kornichuk and his wife Wanda. Alexandre told us that for years Wanda had been determined to have a cow, feeling that it would be their bulwark against food shortages, and he had finally given in. Alexandre laughed as he told us about being slaves to that cow. It was a daily ordeal simply to keep the cow fed, cared for, and milked. Occasionally, the cow would roam off, and they would have to go on retrieval expeditions. Eventually, in total exasperation, Alexandre said the cow had to go. They got rid of the cow, and they didn't starve. In fact, Alexandre said, they both felt liberated from a tremendous burden.

Since I never did get my own cow, I spent a good deal of time looking for a farmer who could supply us with clean raw milk. When I found one, I drove twice a week to the farm to pick up the week's supply. And when we moved to Los Angeles, I was pleased to find that raw certified milk is easily available here.

Until the early 1900s, it was common for dairy cows to have tuberculosis. Also, many people contracted undulant fever (brucellosis) from contaminated milk and fresh cheese due to the unsanitary conditions in dairies. Consequently, pasteurization, a process devised by Louis Pasteur, seemed to solve the problem and became the norm in our country.

The United States Public Health Service defines pasteurization as the process of heating milk to 143° for at least 30 minutes or to 161° for 15 seconds. Pasteur's theories were based upon studies of the heat resistance of *Mycobacterium tuberculosis*, considered one of the most heat-resistant of the monospore-forming microorganisms that may cause disease in human beings. Since such treatment also destroys most of the microorganisms that can cause spoilage, milk thus processed has a longer shelf life.

I suspect that this is one of the reasons most dairies prefer to sell pasteurized milk: raw milk is far more fragile; it remains sweet in the refrigerator for only about four days. The strict rules governing the sanitary conditions and health of the people handling the milk in certified milk plants, as well as the health of the cows, make it much easier to produce pasteurized milk. However, if you live in an area where a dairy is willing to make the extra effort to provide raw certified milk, you are indeed fortunate.

According to the International College of Applied Nutrition, pasteurization not only kills enzymes that make milk digestible and easily absorbed, it destroys 100 percent of the vitamin A, 6 percent of the calcium (and the rest is so altered that the body has difficulty assimilating it), 20 percent of the iodine, 40 percent of the B vitamins, all of the 24 vital trace minerals, most or all of the vitamin C, and 17 percent of the protein.

But it is no longer necessary to pasteurize milk. We now know how to keep a cow healthy, clean, and disease-free. We also have the technology to produce clean raw milk.

Dr. Kurt A. Oster, chief of cardiology at Park City Hospital, Bridgeport, Connecticut, also feels that homogenizing milk (i.e., breaking up the fat globules in milk and dispersing them equally throughout) is harmful because that process reduces the size of the fat particles in the milk, allowing them to be absorbed into the stomach lining in a manner not contemplated by nature. When these fat particles get into the bloodstream, the body sets up a defense mechanism that results in the thickening and hardening of arteries, causing atherosclerosis.

Finally, despite all you have heard to the contrary, drinking low-fat and nonfat pasteurized milk has disadvantages. First the more fat you remove from milk, the less calcium you can assimilate. The butterfat in milk is an integral element in the metabolism of the calcium in milk. And infants and elderly people depend on milk as their main source of calcium. Second, vitamin D, which is fat-soluble, is usually added to pasteurized milk. But by eliminating the butterfat from the milk, the vitamin D is rendered useless.

If milk agrees with you and you like it, you should drink the best—raw certified whole milk. Some people find that yogurt and kefir are easier to digest. But be sure that the yogurt or kefir you consume is made from whole milk.

Norman has always been and probably always will be lean. Recently, however, he has become concerned about putting on weight. Even so, I add milk to his oatmeal or brown rice at breakfast, and make his hot drink with milk. He likes yogurt and eats it three or four times a week. Even more important than being thin is being healthy, I say.

The Wonders of Water

Now we come to water, the most important substance in the human body. Most people do not drink it in adequate amounts. A sufficient level of body fluids is maintained partly by physiological signals that cause the mouth to become dry, creating thirst and encouraging us to drink. If we do not obey these signals and the water level in the body becomes too low, an antidiuretic hormone (vasopressin) is activated, causing water to be reabsorbed into the bloodstream rather than excreted.

Researchers from Oxford and Johns Hopkins have shown that, as the body ages, the kidneys lose their ability to respond to the hormonal signal they receive when a water deficit causes dehydration. The elderly, whether they are in good health or not, will probably not drink enough water.

Norman is no exception. He is so preoccupied with his busy life at UCLA that he sometimes fails to respond to his body's signals. When he comes home after a very hot day and I ask him what kind of a day he had, he will stand there, with his hat still on his head, thinking. As he thinks, he runs his tongue over his lips. It is obvious (at least to me) that he is thirsty. I hand him a glass of water. He drinks it and says, "Thanks. That hit the spot."

I have now decided—since he is an absent-minded professor—to help him remember this important fact of life. Here is how I learned.

Some years ago, I began to feel as if I had sand in my eyes. I consulted an eye doctor in New York City who told me that calcium deposits under my eyelids were causing the trouble; he removed the deposits. A year later, the condition recurred and was corrected the same way. We moved to Los Angeles about that time, and when, a year after that, I again felt as if sand were in my eyes, I went to the Jules Stein Eye Clinic at UCLA. The diagnosis was that my eyes were too dry. The solution was simple: I was advised to buy artificial tears from the pharmacy and to put them into my eyes two or three times a day. I bought the artificial tears and used them to good effect. Eventually, however, I realized that I should be able to make my own tears. I increased my water intake and since that time have had no problem.

Later, when I developed some ulcer symptoms, I discovered that when I drank at least six glasses of water during the day and additional water whenever I awoke during the night, my ulcer symptoms disappeared. My doctor applauds this solution to the problem. He has explained that acid may be generated in the stomach by psychic factors. Moreover, hunger, thoughts of food, the smell of food, and certainly the taste of food all trigger the flow of digestive juices. Thus, a long delay before a meal can mean that there is a lot of acid in an empty stomach. So if you are uncomfortable because a meal is late, drink a glass of water. The water will dilute the acid and rinse the stomach lining.

An adequate supply of water enables us to digest food, maintains normal bodily functions, and allows us to get rid of waste material. Water is no less vital to good health than are protein, vitamins, and minerals. Every cell, every organ in the body needs an adequate supply of this nutrient. Your bones are 25 percent water; your brain and muscles are 75 percent water. Water is necessary to maintain blood volume (our blood is 83 percent water). Increasing liquid intake lowers cholesterol, protects the heart, and lubricates hair, eyes, and skin.

Another reason for drinking water is that it creates a high volume of urine, which keeps the kidneys functioning well—it is easier for kidneys to filter diluted urine than concentrated urine. This is especially important for a person with impaired kidney function. Since about 1 percent of people have a tendency to form kidney stones, with a high intake of water, there is less chance that the stones will form. This is also true of gout, which is caused by an excess of uric acid in the blood. Sodium urate crystals precipitate into joints and tendons, resulting in severe inflammation.

How much water should you drink? It depends on many things—on your size and what you do all day, for instance. Do you live in a hot climate? A big person working in the sun could easily drink a gallon of liquid a day, whereas a small person who physically does little or nothing could use as little as a quart of liquid a day. It is safe to say that the average person should drink at least six to eight glasses of water a day. Even better, drink a glass of water every hour. Soft drinks are undesirable because of the high amount of sugar or sugar substitutes they contain.

When we lived in Connecticut, our water came from our own underground spring. It was wonderful water; we never had any trouble with it. Shortly after we moved to Los Angeles, we read newspaper stories about water pollution in the area, and I started to buy bottled spring water for drinking and cooking. Recently, I had a reverse-osmosis filtering system installed under my kitchen sink. According to the literature, this system filters out the chlorine (which, if ingested for long periods, can cause cancer in some people) but does not filter out those minerals that are necessary for good health. I don't understand how it works, but I am told that at this time reverse osmosis is the most sensible solution to the problem of water pollution.

There are other alternatives: bottled distilled water and a home distillation system. Unfortunately, distilled water contains no minerals, so you may want to compensate with mineral supplements. In any case, distilled water mixes with your body fluids and is transformed into one of the elements of your blood. Distilled water does not taste as good as natural water—it has a "dead" taste—but it is pure. If your local water is inferior and you cannot obtain pure spring water, distilled water is an option.

One word of caution. If a water softener has been installed in your house, make sure that the cold water used for cooking and drinking is not affected by the water-softening process. It is difficult to wash clothes or dishes in hard water because of the minerals, but your heart needs those minerals. When water is softened, the minerals are removed. So, soften the hot water but not the cold.

I am worried about the way we waste water in this country. I believe that unless we change, we will face a dangerous water shortage in the not too distant future.

Dr. John R. Shaeffer and Leonard A. Stevens, in their book *Future Water* (William Morrow, 1983), propose a solution to this problem. They suggest theat we route the sewage from our towns and cities to large reservoirs where it can be treated and used to fertilize and irrigate farms, parks, golf courses, green belts, and the like. The water would then filter down through the soil, which is nature's way of purifying water, and could be routed back into our rivers and streams and used again and again. This would clean up our waterways (and the oceans as well) and would save billions of dollars we now spend on fertilizers.

The method is now being used successfully in many places in the United States. For the last fifty years, for example, a sewage plant located in the middle of Golden Gate Park has supplied irrigation and fertilization for all the trees and plantings in that beautiful park. Pepperdine University in Malibu, California, uses its sewage water to irrigate its lovely campus in the same way.

I hope you feel as strongly as I do about the need to recycle our water and that you will spread the word.

Our Typical Day: From Breakfast to Dinner

BREAKFAST

I suppose the habit of eating breakfast is formed early in life. Some people don't feel like putting food in their mouths before 11:00 A.M. or later. But Norman and I were both brought up in households in which a large breakfast was the only way to start the day. Norman's breakfast these days usually consists of the following:

- Freshly squeezed orange juice or grapefruit juice, *or* a serving of sliced peaches, papaya, banana, or whatever is available.
- A bowl of oatmeal or brown rice and wheat berries with milk and honey.
- Plain yogurt and 1 or 2 slices of whole-wheat bread, *or* 1 egg, soft-boiled, scrambled, or sunny-side up.

- A hot milk drink, consisting of 2 cups of milk, ½ teaspoon of Cafix (a coffee substitute made from roasted grains and figs), ½ teaspoon of blackstrap molasses, and 1 scant teaspoon of honey.
- One or 2 homemade cookies (see p. 132).
- Vitamin supplements.

This is indeed a generous breakfast, and a few words about it may be in order.

Orange juice. In my opinion, there is no substitute for freshly squeezed orange juice. The only thing better is to eat the whole orange, which would provide more fiber. The vitamin C in the fresh fruit and the vitamin A and bioflavonoids in the pulp of the orange, which enhance healing in the body, are not to be found in concentrate or in any other processed form of orange juice.

I find it hard to restrain myself from expressing this opinion when I stand at the check-out counter behind a person whose shopping cart contains a carton labeled "100% orange juice, made from concentrate." I yearn to say, "When you buy orange juice made from concentrate, you are paying a lot of money for water." And yet this is the kind of orange juice most people buy—whatever their circumstances. Evidently, they ask only that the orange juice be conveniently packaged.

Oatmeal. The Quaker Oats Company sells a line of cereals, brand-named "Mother's," that includes rolled oats, and oatmeal with an extra thick flake; oat bran, which nutritionists now claim is the best type of fiber available; and a whole-wheat cereal made from the whole grain. I combine all three when I cook oatmeal. The fiber and nutrition are enhanced, and we think the flavor is better.

If you are preparing food for someone who needs extra nutrition but is unable to eat large amounts at a time, it might be a good idea to add raw egg yolk to the oatmeal. Do not use raw egg white for this purpose (see p. 31).

Yogurt is a wonder food. Culturing milk makes it easy to digest and increases its nutritional value. Some people claim that yogurt aids the immune system and extends the life span.

Stirring brewer's yeast into yogurt is a good way of getting extra nutrition into the diet of a person with a small appetite. It is important to start with small amounts of the yeast— ½ teaspoon, perhaps—and to increase gradually so that the digestive system can adapt to the extra nutrition and your patient can get used to the taste. We like the taste of Plus Products' Super Yeast (Formula 300). Also, adding wheat germ, granular lecithin, blackstrap molasses, cut-up dates, or fresh fruit can provide variety and additional food value to yogurt.

Blackstrap molasses (Plantation brand) is another nutritious marvel. It is an excellent source of iron in a form that is easily assimilated by the body. It is also a good source of calcium, potassium, and other trace minerals. In *Through the Looking-Glass*, Alice speaks of a special treat, "treacle on a slice of bread." Treacle is the uncrystallized syrup produced in the sugar-refining process. It has been used medicinally for hundreds of years, according to the *Shorter Oxford English Dictionary*. Blackstrap molasses is today's version of treacle.

Whole-wheat bread. One of the best ways to provide good nutrition for your family is to bake bread. Thirty years ago I found a recipe in the *New York*

Times, and I have been using it ever since—with slight variations (see p. 112).

Recently, Norman indicated that he wanted to cut down on the amount of food he eats because he has begun to put on weight. I made the same suggestion to him that I just made to you: sprinkle some wheat germ on the yogurt or eggs instead of eating a slice of bread. Whenever weight is a concern, I think it's better to cut down on the quantity—not the quality—of the food you eat.

Eggs. If I had my way, as mentioned earlier, Norman would eat two eggs for breakfast every morning. So far, I have not been able to persuade him to eat even one egg a day.

The best way to prepare an egg is to soft-boil or hard-boil it. Fifteen percent of the thiamin and riboflavin is lost when the egg is cooked out of the shell.

Hot milk drink. Cafix, an instant beverage imported from West Germany, is made from roasted malt, chicory, barley, rye, shredded beet roots, and figs; I buy it in the health-food store. When I prepare Cafix, I add some blackstrap molasses to it. Although Cafix's taste is pleasant in itself, more importantly, it will cover the taste of the molasses, which is the most valuable ingredient in the hot drink. However, a little blackstrap molasses goes a long way: 1 teaspoonful a day is adequate, unless you are constipated; 1 or 2 tablespoons will cure any case of constipation.

A word of warning about honey. A common practice among unscrupulous honey producers is to feed the bees sugar or shopworn candy to speed up production. Honey produced this way is no better than the materials it is made from. Read the label on the container, and try to find honey that is marked "made by the bees from the flower nectar," "organically produced," or "uncooked and unfiltered."

Homemade cookies. Norman likes to have 1 or 2 cookies with his hot milk drink. I make two or three different kinds (see p. 132).

Vitamin supplements. Many people have asked me what vitamin supplements Norman and I take. I think it is a good idea to take a reliable vitamin-mineral supplement in order to get a balanced formula. For many years, I have given my family Omni-Plex, a complete multivitamin and multimineral supplement with amino acids, enzymes, and other substances. According to the label on the bottle, this supplement is made from high-quality natural ingredients, without synthetic binders and fillers, and without the use of toxic chemical solvents, starch, and sugar. I order Omni-Plex by mail from Essential Organics, P.O. Box 325, Organic Park, Derry, NH 03038; phone: (603) 432–5022.

We occasionally take extra vitamin C, beta carotene, lecithin capsules, vitamin E, zinc, and magnesium; I take 2 dolomite tablets a day.

Norman has no particular fondness for pills—even vitamin pills—and believes that a well-rounded diet provides the vitamins he needs. I recognize the logic of his argument but feel that the problems of modern living, with its smog, car exhaust, industrial pollutants, insecticides—to say nothing of occupational stress and emotional tensions—require a degree of compensating care. We have compromised on vitamins. He now takes four vitamin pills at breakfast including a multivitamin-multimineral tablet.

During the day, when Norman is at home, I take every opportunity to give him some kind of nutritious food or drink. At 11:00 A.M. and at about 4:00 P.M., he eats an apple or a banana. If he is working at his UCLA office, when he comes home he has a glass of borscht, carrot juice, or water.

LUNCH

Compared to breakfast, lunch is a fairly light meal when we are home. I try to have a good supply of fresh vegetables on hand so that I can make a thick soup or prepare a plate of cooked and raw vegetables. There is nothing Norman likes better for lunch than a couple ears of corn (when in season) or a baked potato with some kind of vegetable topping, and one or two other vegetables such as peas, beans, carrots, zucchini, tomatoes.

A baked potato is a small, self-contained supermarket. One potato provides 35 percent of the adult daily requirement of vitamin C. It is superior to other food crops in the quality of its protein, and the ratio of that protein to carbohydrates is higher in a potato than in many cereals and other roots and tubers. In terms of nutritional balance—protein, amino acids, minerals, and vitamins—the potato ranks second only to the egg. As it helps meet all of our daily nutritional needs, it also provides us with a good supply of fiber. A wide range of toppings can add delicious variety, the possibilities limited only by our imagination. Sweet potatoes, too, are an excellent source for many minerals and beta carotene.

A few toppings for baked potatoes, sweet or white:

- Chopped fresh tomato, onion, and yellow squash or zucchini, seasoned with Vege-Sal and sweet basil, and cooked slowly in a small amount of sweet butter in a covered saucepan. Do not add water.

- Cooked lentils or split peas combined with chopped onions and mushrooms that have been sautéed in a little sweet butter.
- Fresh string beans or peas or both, with carrots, spinach, or Swiss chard, guacamole (see p. 69), cottage cheese or yogurt, mixed with chopped red pepper and red onion.

I usually serve a green vegetable with the potato or a side dish of guacamole, cottage cheese, or yogurt.

You will notice that I recommend Vege-Sal for seasoning. This product contains earth and sea-salt crystals, soybean extract, yeast concentrate, celery, carrots, spinach, parsley, onion, alfalfa, beet, watercress, celery root, dill, lettuce, and Pacific sea greens. Used instead of salt, it adds a nice flavor to everything. In fact, a little Vege-Sal and some unrefined sesame oil make a wonderful salad dressing.

Once a week Norman plays golf with three of his friends. They usually eat lunch while they play. Norman carries with him a thermos of thick vegetable soup and some whole-wheat bread or crackers. Because he felt uncomfortable enjoying the soup while his buddies munched on hot dogs available on the course, I now provide four thermoses of soup—one for each man in the foursome.

On Saturday and Sunday mornings, Norman and I usually play tennis doubles. Before we go on the court, I start a pot of soup. Some split peas or lentils and barley in a pot of water or chicken broth with some cut-up carrots, celery, and potato make a good base for a thick soup. I put the pot over very low heat and let the soup cook slowly. By the time we finish playing, we are ready for lunch and all I need to do is add some fresh green vegetables to the pot a few minutes before I serve the soup.

One Saturday I made a red-bean soup (see pp. 78–80), which is one of Norman's favorites. Then I served broiled sea bass on brown rice, topped with a sauce of tomatoes and onions cooked in a little butter.

One Sunday, after our tennis game, I gave Norman cabbage salad (see pp. 119–120) and a bowl of split-pea and barley soup (see p. 76) for lunch. Afterward, I decided to count the number of vegetables and grains included in that one meal. I was surprised to find that the total was fifteen: the salad contained six; the soup consisted of rice, barley, split peas, carrots, celery, onions, string beans, and peas; and Norman ate the soup with a slice of whole-wheat bread.

As you can see, I am in favor of a wide variety of vegetables. Recent reports from nutrition research centers confirm this opinion. Heart patients, as well as people who are interested in maintaining good health, would do well to follow the advice of the National Cancer Institute, given in a report of a recent study (1986). The study involved 763 lung-cancer patients in New Jersey who were asked about their usual intake of those foods that provide most of the vitamin A in the U.S. diet and about their use of vitamin supplements. The purpose of the study was to determine whether dietary intake of carotenoids influenced the risk of lung cancer. Carotenoids are substances like beta carotene that are found in plant foods and that the body converts to vitamin A.

When the patients and controls were evaluated according to consumption of carotenoids, researchers found that those in the lowest fourth of estimated consumption had about a 30-percent greater chance of getting lung cancer than those in the highest fourth of estimated consumption. Although the study found that the greatest protection against lung cancer was afforded by a diet high in dark-green, yellow and orange fruits and vegetables and by a diet high in carotene, and that no apparent protection against the disease is offered by the intake of preformed active vitamin A, these recommendations can be applied to anyone interested in a good diet.

For the last three years, I have been concerned about the methods used in raising chickens and in producing eggs commercially. Earlier in this book, I discussed eggs and recommended that you try to buy fertile eggs because they are better for you and more likely to have been produced under healthier conditions than commercially produced sterile eggs.

Since I often use chicken broth when I make soup, I should explain that I buy chickens from a reliable health-food store that claims to deal only with producers who raise their fowls in a natural environment and give them chemical-free, high-quality feed. I buy the whole chicken, preferably a roaster, rather than chicken parts (I want to see *all* of the bird), and I ask the butcher to examine it very carefully for bruises or sores or broken bones.

Nobel laureate Dr. Francis Peyton Rous, of the Rockefeller Institute for Medical Research, has said (in Virginia Livingston-Wheeler, *The Conquest of Cancer* [New York, 1984], pp. 113–119) that 95 percent of the chickens for sale in New York City are cancerous and that the material that he called a "tumor agent" was definitely transmissible to humans.

Although no one can offer total reassurance, it is possible to reduce the risk when purchasing poultry. Learn to know the difference between a bruise and a sore. Bruises can be caused by rough handling in the process of removing the feathers; sores may be indications of a systemic disorder. Reject any chicken with either a bruise or a sore.

Make sure that your chicken is thoroughly cooked (that is, to an internal temperature of 180° Fahrenheit). Be especially cautious about chickens broiled on a barbecue or cooked in a wok—they may be only partially cooked on the inside. Also, choose your butcher as carefully as you would an in-law (if you had your choice)—find someone you can trust.

Remove as much fat as possible from poultry prior to cooking, since pesticides and other fat-soluble agrichemicals accumulate in fatty tissue. Avoid eating the liver and kidneys of commercially grown animals, since these organs may contain a high amount of drug residues.

As a result of the increasing publicity about the dangers of eating poultry, Norman and I avoid eating chicken at large public dinners. We find ourselves moving ever closer to a diet consisting of vegetables, fruits, legumes, grains, seeds, dairy products, eggs, and fish. We are not bereft, however. The variety of taste and texture within those categories is great and satisfying.

DINNER

Looking at Norman today—athletic, strong, healthy— I find it difficult to believe that as a child he was fragile and sickly, with little appetite. His mother told me that she used a number of tricks to persuade him to eat. For instance, since she knew he loved corn on the cob, she would give it to him as a reward after he had eaten the rest of his dinner. As he grew older, he became stronger and taller, and his appetite improved—the result, perhaps, of his active interest in sports, especially in baseball. But his mother still made him eat his entire meal before she would serve the corn.

After we were married, I offered to give him the corn early in the meal; Norman enthusiastically endorsed the idea. And that is how I have served it ever since.

When we lived in Connecticut, I grew wonderful corn. (That was even the name of it: Harris' Wonderful Corn.) Now, in Los Angeles, I have found a farm not too far from our home where corn is picked daily, so it is sweet and fresh and almost as good as the corn I grew. Norman tries to limit himself to one ear per meal because he is concerned about putting on too much weight.

Borrowing some of Mom's tactics, we always have a cabbage salad as a first course at dinner, even though Norman is not overly fond of it. But I know he will eat it when he is hungry, and it is an important source of fiber in his diet. I suspect that if I were to serve the cabbage salad after the main course, some of it would remain on the plate.

When we lived in New Canaan, we always had a large chicken dinner at three o'clock Sunday afternoon, and Norman would invite his friends to come out from New York for the day. I remember one Sunday dinner in particular. Andy Holt, then president of Tennessee State University, was our visitor. At that time, Shigeko Sasamori, one of the Hiroshima Maidens, was living with us. Norman was telling Andy about our flock of Rhode Island Red chickens. He claimed that each egg was produced at a cost of at least 50 cents. Shigeko explained that the reason for the high cost was that each egg contained at least two yolks, sometimes more. Andy asked for proof, and Shigeko ran out to the chicken yard and came back with a huge egg. When I opened the egg in a soup bowl, Andy almost fell off his chair. Out came four yolks.

Shigeko lived with us for more than fifteen years in New Canaan; she and her son Norman are considered members of our family. As a result, we have added many Japanese foods to our diet, and everyone in the family is adept at using chopsticks.

Dinner, as mentioned earlier, begins with cabbage salad (see p. 119). Sometimes, to provide variety, I whirl it in the blender, turning it into a kind of gazpacho. Then I serve the corn, if I have it on hand. If Norman has not had soup for lunch, I will serve a small bowl of split-pea and barley soup, white-bean soup, or chicken-with-rice soup. The main course might be a small serving of fish (salmon, sea bass, trout, or whitefish) and a vegetable such as peas, asparagus, spinach, green beans, or eggplant cooked with tomato and onion (see p. 109). Often, we have a meatless meal—brown rice and beans or tofu and vegetables.

When I make rice, I add some wheat berries and cook them together until the rice is done, leaving the wheat berries a little crunchy. I usually make more than I need so that Norman can have some for breakfast the following morning. And I do the same with beans because Norman loves beans of all kinds: red, white, black, chickpeas, adzukis—it doesn't matter what kind they are or how they are prepared. Bean soup Mexican style, bean salad, even just plain shelled boiled beans—he likes them all. So, quite often I add beans to the dinner menu because it is such a good source of fiber and minerals. Also, the combination of brown rice and beans provides all the amino acids necessary to form a complete protein.

In case you are not familiar with adzuki beans, I recommend them. They are very small red beans from Japan. Good for sprouting and cooking, they cook in a much shorter time than regular beans and can be added to soups and salads. You can find them in most health-food stores.

Including tofu (bean curd) in the diet helps to bring down the cholesterol count because it is made from soybeans. It is not necessary to cook tofu. Just before serving fish or vegetables, I add tofu to the pot so that the tofu will get heated through and take on some of the flavor of the fish or vegetables since it has little flavor of its own.

Like most people, we have sharply reduced our intake of red meat. Recent research shows that people who eat fish regularly are less likely to suffer heart attacks. It has been found that certain fish oils contain substances called omega-3 long-chain fatty acids that tend to induce favorable changes in the blood. One of these fatty acids, eicosapentaenoic acid (EPA), is found in salt-water marine animals and fish but not in land animals. Salmon and mackerel are especially rich sources of these fatty acids. Fish oil has numerous beneficial physiological effects, including the reduction of blood triglycerides, blood pressure, and platelet clumping. There is also evidence that fish oil has antiinflammatory and antiarthritic properties.

However, these benefits are not as clear-cut in canned fish. Although omega-3 fatty acids have not been destroyed by canning, canned salmon and mackerel have been found to contain mutagens (substances capable of inducing changes in the DNA of living cells; they are considered to be carcinogenic).

Since mutagens are not present in the unprocessed raw fish, it is probable that they are introduced in the canning process.

Sometimes we save dessert for later in the evening. Then we have a small bowl of apples stewed in honey with plums or raisins (see p. 128), or a Bartlett pear stewed in honey with a cinnamon stick (see p. 129), or some other kind of stewed or fresh fruit, custard (see p. 125), or rice pudding (see p. 124).

Travel and Eating Out

Travel is an important part of Norman's life. Whenever he goes off on a two- or three-day trip, I slip a few apples and other goodies into his suitcase, knowing that he enjoys a snack. Norman thought I was overdoing it, however, when he was packing to go to Korea to report on the Korean War for the American Broadcasting Company. I knew that he would be traveling in an army plane, and I thought it would be a good idea to have some extra food along. So I buried some small cans of chicken, salmon, sardines, and whole-wheat crackers among the socks and handkerchiefs. When Norman noticed what I was doing, he tossed the cans out, saying that his luggage would be overweight; but before he took off, the cans were back in again.

As it turned out, my concern was justified. On the flight to Korea from Japan the army plane ran into bad weather and had to force-land, pancaking down in a rice field about 50 miles from the airfield outside Seoul. The captain went off to find help, and eight men huddled under the wing in the heavy rain. There was nothing to eat. Hoping I had been more successful than he had thought, Norman poked into the corners of his suitcase and happily came across the edible treasures. Since it was almost five hours before a rescue party arrived, the food could not have been more appreciated.

When Norman and I travel together by plane, we try to order a vegetarian meal, which usually consists of a salad, mixed hot vegetables, some cheese, and fresh fruit—a simple but adequate meal.

Some years ago in the Soviet Union, we flew from Moscow to Irkutsk in Siberia. Lunch was served in a brown paper bag, which the airline attendant tossed to passengers as she walked down the aisle. Inside the bag were a piece of cold roasted chicken, two slices of dark bread, a wedge of cheese, a fresh cucumber, a tomato, and an apple. We thought it a wholesome meal.

In 1987, Norman and I went to Hiroshima, where he was awarded the first Kiyoshi Tanimoto Peace Prize. Norman was awarded the prize because of his work in providing medical care and rehabilitation for the survivors of the Hiroshima and Nagasaki bombings. We stayed at the ANA Hiroshima Hotel. The food was excellent. My only complaint (and I thought it best not to complain) was the lack of whole-wheat bread and brown rice. But I was keenly interested to learn that no Japanese breakfast is complete without a salad. They have some kind of tool that makes it possible to shred red cabbage, red onion, green pepper, and radishes so finely that it is like eating crisp air. The Japanese salad dressing is a vinaigrette made with toasted sesame seeds. I haven't quite succeeded in duplicating the uniquely subtle taste of this delicious salad, but it is a challenge I find difficult to resist.

When Norman is traveling and I stay home, I must

confess I do not go to great lengths to prepare food for myself. At those times, I eat very simply: a baked potato, cottage cheese, raw vegetables. But I force myself to eat nutritious foods in order to stay healthy. (I think one of the greatest favors people can do for their loved ones is to spare them the burden of being sick.) Since, in recent years, Norman has cut down on long air trips and has rearranged his life so he is home more often, my diet has improved accordingly, as a by-product of my efforts on his behalf.

However, he still gives quite a few lectures locally, to which we travel by car. I always bring along a basket of fruit, Dofino, Havarti or Jarlsberg cheese, whole-wheat bread or crackers, homemade brownies or cookies, or any other nutritious snacks that I happen to have in the house, such as raisins, nuts, whole-wheat fig cookies. We have learned that nothing is better than a handful of raisins and peanuts or almonds to provide quick energy, preventing drowsiness at the wheel.

When we must stay overnight in a hotel, we have learned to make do with the best of what is offered. But we do try to order fresh, unprocessed food whenever possible. At breakfast, for instance, if we have a choice between half a grapefruit and "fresh" orange juice, we choose the grapefruit; the orange juice is likely to be reconstituted from concentrate. Instead of a small box of corn flakes or some other processed concoction, we ask for hot oatmeal or another whole-grain cooked cereal. A sensible choice for breakfast away from home might be two soft-boiled eggs with buttered whole-wheat toast and a bowl of yogurt. Many so-called whole-wheat breads are made partly with white flour. Rye bread is almost 100-percent white flour. Even bran muffins are sometimes made with white flour. But these are the hazards of travel.

At lunch or dinner, avoid creamed soups because the thickening agent is usually white flour. Choose a fresh vegetable soup, if possible. For the same reason, it is best to avoid fish or meat dipped in batter and fried or served with a cream sauce. The best choices are roasted, broiled or grilled fish or meats and fresh vegetables. You are fortunate if the menu offers a spinach salad with cheese, cottage cheese and fresh fruit, broiled salmon and fresh cooked spinach, or a baked potato and a broiled lamb chop.

If possible, order fresh fruit for dessert. Ice cream is an extremely high-fat, high-sugar food, no matter what the sweetener is, and should be avoided, especially if you are sedentary or overweight, or if you have heart or circulatory problems. The FDA allows over 100 ingredients in ice cream, including chemicals for thickening, stabilizing, and emulsifying. Ice-cream manufacturers are not even required to tell you if the coloring agent is natural or artificial. Some of the chemicals used in making ice cream are also used for making plastic, shoes, and paint thinner.

When we go to public dinners, I think it prudent to give Norman a bowl of soup and some bread before we leave. Sometimes it is 9:00 P.M. before people are actually served—too long a stretch for a person who has had an early breakfast and a light lunch. It makes it possible for him to resist eating the fancy hors d'oeuvres made with white flour.

We have learned to avoid the following:

- All sodas. They have no nutritional value. Moreover, they often contain caffeine, food colorings, phosphates, and saccharin, all of which are dangerous.
- All beverages and foods that contain NutraSweet or other chemical sweetener.
- Cured meats such as corned beef, salami, bacon, sausages, hot dogs, since they often contain sugar, sodium phosphate and sodium phosphite, colorings, and other chemicals.

You might think I am being fanatical, and you'd be right. But I am determined not to be a widow, and I can see that Norman has never been in better shape. He has recovered rapidly from broken bones due to falls on the tennis court, and from the usual sprains and bruises that accompany an active life. His doctors are amazed at his recuperative powers, which they say they would find remarkable in a man in his twenties. Dr. David Cannom, his cardiologist, marvels at Norman's electrocardiogram readings. They show that much of the damage caused by Norman's massive heart attack in 1980 has been reversed. I know that a good deal of this improvement is due to Norman's positive attitude. But I am also sure that the good food I have given Norman during the years since his heart attack have helped make his dramatic recovery possible.

Entertaining

Some years ago, Norman and I attended a dinner in New York City at the home of Ambassador Rossides of Cyprus. Mrs. Rossides was concerned about her husband's health and made sure he ate nothing but foods that were good for him. On this occasion, he had brown rice and fresh vegetables, but the rest of us were served "regular food." Mrs. Rossides probably did not wish to impose her dietary regime on her guests. But I do not hold such reservations. Everyone who comes to our house knows that whatever I serve Norman is good for them, too.

Norman is always trying to spare me the work of cooking when we entertain guests, and often urges me to hire a caterer. I am willing to get whatever help I need to serve the food and drink and to clean up afterward, but I insist on doing the cooking myself. I enjoy making unusual combinations of dishes and serving them to our friends. Many people are not familiar with lentils, adzuki beans, fava beans, buckwheat groats (kasha), or wild rice, and have never tasted celery root, rutabaga, or turnip greens, all of which are delicious and nutritious.

For a dinner party for twelve last New Year's Eve, I roasted four fresh ducks. With this, I served my usual cabbage salad, wild rice, and the three-vegetable dish known as "red, white, and green," consisting of red sweet peppers, cauliflower, and fresh string beans (see p. 107). I also served homemade mango chutney, which goes well with poultry and lamb (see p. 103). It was a simple meal, easy to prepare and everyone seemed to enjoy it. Many of our guests returned to the buffet table for second helpings.

In the summer, I often poach a whole salmon as a main dish and serve it hot with wild or brown rice, one or two vegetables, and a salad. As a first course, I serve cold beet soup made with fresh beets, honey, fresh lemon juice, and yogurt (see p. 81).

Now that our children are grown and out of the house and we have made many new friends in Los Angeles, we do far more entertaining than we did in Connecticut. I enjoy making each meal—with or without guests—as heathful and, of course, as tasty as possible. I know that Norman appreciates my efforts. And I think our friends do, too, because they are constantly asking me for the recipes for the dishes I serve. Many of these are now included in this book.

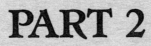

PART 2

Hors d'Oeuvres

YOGURT DIP

6 walnut halves
1 clove garlic, peeled
1 tablespoon olive oil
1 cup plain yogurt

¼ cup peeled, finely
   diced cucumber
½ teaspoon fresh
   lemon juice

In a blender or food processor, blend the walnuts, garlic, and olive oil. In a serving bowl, combine the mixture with the yogurt, cucumber, and lemon juice. Chill the dip, and serve it with raw vegetables or whole-wheat crackers.

Yield: about 1 cup.

GUACAMOLE

This recipe will also serve 3 or 4 as a side dish.

2 or 3 avocados
Juice of 1 lemon
1 red onion, peeled
   and finely minced

1 clove garlic, peeled
   and finely minced
Vege-Sal, to taste

Peel the avocados. Cut them in half, remove the pit, and place them in a bowl. Add the lemon juice to the bowl, and mash the avocados with a fork. Stir in the onion, garlic, and Vege-Sal, refrigerate the guacamole until time to serve, and serve it with whole-wheat crackers.

(*Note:* The guacamole should not be refrigerated for more than 1 hour.)

Yield: 4 to 6 servings.

STUFFED EGGS WITH TOASTED SESAME SEEDS

6 hard-boiled eggs, shelled and halved lengthwise	1 tablespoon chopped parsley
¼ cup plain yogurt	¼ teaspoon dried marjoram
¼ cup toasted sesame seeds (see Note, below)	Vege-Sal, to taste
	Toasted sesame seeds for garnish

Remove the yolks from the egg halves, and mash the yolks in a bowl. Add the other ingredients, except the garnish, to the yolks, and stir the mixture to blend. Fill the egg-white halves with the yolk mixture, and garnish the eggs with toasted sesame seeds.

(*Note:* To toast sesame seeds, place the seeds in a small pan over low heat. Stir them occasionally until they are golden brown. Remember, unhulled seeds are more nutritious than hulled seeds—the hulls are full of minerals.)

Yield: 12 stuffed eggs.

CHEDDAR ROUNDS

1 cup grated sharp
    Cheddar
½ cup (1 stick) sweet
    butter, melted
½ teaspoon Vege-Sal
    or soy sauce

1 pinch cayenne
½ cup whole-wheat
    flour
    (approximately)

Preheat the oven to 400°. In a bowl, combine the cheese, butter, Vege-Sal or soy sauce, and cayenne. Add the flour gradually, mixing the ingredients until the dough is of the right consistency to be handled. Shape the dough into 24 small balls, place the balls on a buttered cookie sheet, flatten the balls, and bake the rounds for about 5 minutes or until they are golden brown.

Yield: 24 rounds.

CHICKEN-LIVER PÂTÉ

1 egg, washed
1 cup water
1 stalk celery, finely
    diced
1–2 small carrots,
    scrubbed and
    diced
1 tablespoon millet
Vege-Sal, to taste
1 large onion, peeled
    and diced
1 tablespoon sweet
    butter

4–5 chicken livers, cut
    up
1 handful fresh
    parsley, washed
    and chopped
1 teaspoon freshly
    ground black
    pepper
2 tablespoons unrefined
    sesame oil
½ cup toasted wheat
    germ
1 teaspoon brewer's
    yeast

Place the egg in a small saucepan with the water, and, over high heat, bring the water to a boil. Reduce the heat, and simmer the egg for 12 minutes. Remove the egg, and reserve the water. Peel the egg, and set it aside. Cook the celery, carrot(s), and millet in the reserved water until the vegetables are barely tender. Add the Vege-Sal.

In a frying pan, sauté the onion in the butter until the onion is slightly browned. Add the chicken livers, and cook them until they are done.

Strain the vegetables and millet, reserving the water, and combine them in a blender with the livers and onion. Add to the mixture the parsley, pepper, sesame oil, wheat germ, brewer's yeast, and enough of the reserved water to make a smooth paste. Remove the pâté from the blender. Chop the reserved hard-boiled egg, and add it to the liver paste. Chill, garnish, and serve the pâté with whole-wheat crackers.

Yield: 3 cups.

PIROSHKI

I make piroshki only for special occasions, such as when we entertain the delegates of the Soviet-American Writers' Conference, of which Norman is the co-chairman. It takes time. But most people like them, so it is worth the effort. With the piroshki, which are served warm, I serve cold beet soup in small punch cups (see p. 81).

DOUGH

1 package dry yeast
1 cup warm
    (between 105°
    and 115°) milk
4 cups stone-ground
    whole-wheat
    flour
    (approximately)
1 teaspoon Vege-Sal
2 teaspoons honey
3 eggs, slightly
    beaten
1 cup (2 sticks)
    sweet butter,
    melted and
    cooled

FILLING

1 onion, peeled and
    chopped
1/4 cup (1/2 stick)
    sweet butter,
    melted
3 cups chopped or
    ground leftover
    cooked
    chicken, lamb,
    or beef, *or*
    chicken livers,
    or buckwheat
    groats (kasha),
    or any kind of
    cooked
    vegetable
2 hard-boiled eggs,
    chopped
2 tablespoons
    minced parsley
Vege-Sal, to taste
Freshly ground
    pepper, to taste

2 egg whites, slightly
    beaten

To make the dough, dissolve the yeast in the milk. Stir in 1 cup of the flour. Let the starter rise in a warm place for about 1 hour.

Add the Vege-Sal, honey, eggs, melted butter, and the remaining flour to the yeast mixture. Mix the ingredients well, and knead the dough until it becomes smooth and elastic—for 8 to 10 minutes. Form the dough into a ball, and place it in a buttered bowl. Cover the dough, and let it rise in a warm place for 3 to 4 hours or until it has doubled in bulk and is springy to the touch.

Meanwhile, make the filling. In a saucepan, sauté the onion in the butter. Add the remaining filling ingredients, and combine them well. Correct the seasonings. Set the filling aside.

After the dough has risen, take off a piece of it about as big as your fist. On a floured surface, roll the dough out until it is ¼ inch thick. Cut out circles of dough, using a 3½-inch round cookie cutter or jar lid. Elongate each circle with a rolling pin. Place about 1 tablespoon of the reserved filling down the middle of each piece of dough. Dip your finger in the egg white, and paint the edges of each oval with the white. Fold the piroshki lengthwise, pressing the edges of the dough together. Set the pastries on a lightly buttered and floured cookie sheet. Repeat this process until all the dough and filling have been used up.

Preheat the oven to 400°.

Let the piroshki rise for 15 minutes. Brush egg white on the top of the piroshki, and form each pastry into a crescent by gently pulling the points toward one another. Bake the piroshki for 15 minutes at 400°; then lower the heat to 300°, and bake the pastries for another 20 minutes.

Yield: about 48 piroshki.

Soups

LENTIL SOUP

1 clove garlic, minced
1 onion, peeled and
   minced
2 tablespoons sweet
   butter
2 tablespoons
   unrefined sesame
   oil

1 cup lentils
4 cups chicken broth
1 carrot, scrubbed and
   sliced
1 stalk celery, minced
1 bay leaf

In a large soup pot, sauté the garlic and onion in the butter and sesame oil until the vegetables are golden brown. Add the lentils, chicken broth, carrot, celery, and bay leaf to the pot. Cook the soup for 1 hour. Remove the bay leaf, and serve the soup.

Yield: 4 to 5 servings.

SPLIT-PEA AND BARLEY SOUP

Leftover lamb or chicken or vegetables can be added to this soup, if desired.

4 cups water
1 heaping tablespoon barley
2 heaping tablespoons split peas
1 potato, scrubbed and diced
2 stalks celery, diced
1 large onion, scrubbed and finely diced

2 carrots, peeled and diced
Vege-Sal, to taste
½ teaspoon fresh or dried basil
1 handful fresh string beans *or* 1 cup peas

In a large saucepan over high heat, bring the water to a boil. Add to the pan all the ingredients, except for the string beans or peas, in the order listed. Lower the heat, and simmer the soup until the barley is tender—for about 30 minutes. A few minutes before serving, add the string beans or peas to the soup.

Yield: 3 to 4 servings.

SATURDAY SOUP

2 shoulder lamb chops,
    fat removed
2 pieces
    (approximately ½
    pound) beef
    shank
6–8 cups water
½ cup lentils
2 tablespoons barley
1 onion, peeled and
    chopped

1 stalk celery, chopped
2 carrots, scrubbed
    and diced
2 cups water
1 cup fresh peas
Vege-Sal, to taste
½ teaspoon fresh or
    dried basil

In a soup pot, simmer the lamb and beef in the 6 to 8 cups of water for about 2 hours or until the meat is tender. In the meantime, combine the lentils, barley, onion, celery, and carrots in a small saucepan with the 2 cups of water. Cover the pan, and cook the mixture over low heat until the barley is tender—about 30 minutes.

Strain the meat broth, reserving the broth. Remove the meat from the bones, and set it aside, discarding the bones. Return the meat broth to the soup pot, and combine the broth with the cooked vegetable-lentil-barley mixture, and with the reserved meat. Add the fresh peas to pot, and bring the soup to a boil. Add the Vege-Sal and basil. Cook the peas until they are tender—for about 4 minutes. Serve the soup in large soup bowls.

Yield: 4 to 6 servings.

FISH SOUP

½ pound fillet of sole
1 tablespoon soy sauce
1 tablespoon sherry
2 tablespoons
    unrefined sesame
    oil
6 cups chicken *or* fish
    broth
8 tablespoons raw
    brown rice
½ cup celery, diced

½ cup minced onion
½ cup diced carrots
¼ teaspoon freshly
    ground pepper
3 scallions (both green
    and white parts),
    finely sliced

Cut the fish into inch-long strips about ½ inch wide. Mix the fish with the soy sauce, sherry, and sesame oil. Place the fish in the refrigerator.

Meanwhile, in a large saucepan, bring the broth to a boil, stir in the rice, cover the pan, and cook the rice over low heat for 45 minutes. Add the celery, onion, carrots, and pepper to the pan. Cook the vegetables, covered, for 5 minutes. Add the marinated fish to the saucepan, and cook the soup 10 minutes or longer. Before serving, sprinkle the soup with the scallions.

Yield: 4 to 5 servings.

RED-BEAN SOUP

This recipe can be used with other kinds of beans. I make this soup every Thursday for the "golfing foursome." Their praises were louder than usual when I added bits of cooked lamb to the recipe. Since I must fill four pint-sized thermoses, I increase this recipe by adding more fresh tomatoes (or water) than called for.

When I started to make this soup, I was inspired to use fresh tomatoes instead of additional water because I was, at the time, up to my eyes in tomatoes. Since we do not have a good garden site at our home in the craggy canyons overlooking Los Angeles, I've taken to growing vegetables in pots and tubs, and the results are rewarding. We have sweet peppers, zucchinis, onions, potatoes, turnips, beets, Swiss chard, beans, peas, and often more tomatoes than I can handle. Our bumper crops are due partly, I believe, to the fact that I compost my kitchen vegetable garbage and put some of the compost in the bottom of each pot.

In order to preserve the tomatoes from my harvest, I put them (washed) in the freezer, whole. When they are frozen solid, I store them in plastic bags in the freezer. These tomatoes cannot be used in salads, but they are excellent for cooking and in soups.

4 cups dried red
kidney beans
3 heaping tablespoons
green split peas
6–8 cups water
1 large onion, peeled
and chopped
2 stalks celery, finely
diced

6–8 large fresh
tomatoes, diced
3 large carrots,
scrubbed and
diced
2 tablespoons chopped
fresh or dried basil
2 tablespoons chopped
parsley
Vege-Sal, to taste

In a large soup pot, cook the beans and split peas in the water for approximately 2 hours or until the beans and peas are tender. In a second pot, over low heat, combine the onion, celery, tomatoes, and carrots, and cook them slowly in their own juices for 20 to 30 minutes. Add the vegetables to the beans and split peas. Since this makes a thick soup, keep it over very low heat to prevent scorching. Just before serving, add the basil, parsley, and Vege-Sal to the soup.

Yield: 8 or more servings.

CHAWAN MUSHI (CHICKEN-BROTH CUSTARD)

Norman and I first tasted this custard soup in Hiroshima. And our "adopted" daughter Shigeko Sasamori, who lived with us for more than twenty-five years, taught me how to make it.

5 eggs, slightly beaten
6 cups cold seasoned
    chicken broth
Bite-sized pieces of
    fresh raw chicken
    meat *or* raw
    white-fleshed fish

6 fresh spinach leaves,
    stems removed
    and torn into
    several pieces

In a bowl, add the eggs to the broth, and stir the ingredients well. Place 2 or 3 pieces of chicken or fish and 2 or 3 pieces of spinach in each of 6 custard cups. Pour the egg-broth mixture into the cups. Place the cups in a steamer or a pan containing about 2 inches of water. Cover the cups. Simmer the water gently for about 10 minutes or until the custard is set. Serve the chawan mushi either hot or cold.

Yield: 6 servings.

FRESH PEA SOUP

4 pounds fresh peas, shelled (reserve the pods)
6 cups water
2 tablespoons split peas
1 onion, peeled and finely minced
1 stalk celery, finely minced

1 carrot, scrubbed and finely minced
1 egg yolk, lightly beaten
½ cup milk
2 tablespoons finely chopped parsley

Rinse the pea pods, and put them in a soup kettle. Add the water, and bring it to a boil. Cook the pods for a few minutes. Discard the pods. Add the split peas to the pea-pod water, and boil the split peas until they are almost tender—about 20 minutes. Add the onion, celery, and carrot, and bring the soup to a boil. Add the shelled fresh peas, and bring the soup to a boil again. Just before serving, stir the egg yolk into the milk, and add this mixture gradually to the soup. Sprinkle each serving with the parsley.

Yield: 4 to 6 servings.

BEET SOUP (BORSCHT)

This cold soup can be served in a bowl with a hot boiled potato (Russian style) or as a cold drink. On a summer evening, I serve it in punch cups as an appetizer when we have dinner guests. And there is nothing Norman likes better when he comes home from the office on a hot day than a tall, cold glass of borscht. (*Note:* If the beet tops are fresh and crisp, remove the stems, wash the leaves thoroughly, cut the leaves up, and cook them in a small amount of water in a covered saucepan. Beet tops are as nutritious as beets and are delicious.)

1 bunch medium-sized beets, tops removed	**2 tablespoons honey**
	Vege-Sal, to taste
	3–4 cups plain yogurt
4 cups water	
Juice of 1 lemon	

Scrub the beets thoroughly to remove all the sand. Add the beets and the water to a pressure cooker or to a large covered pot and cook the beets until they are tender—about 12 minutes for the pressure cooker and about 30 minutes for the pot. Allow the beets to cool, and remove their skins with a paper towel. Cut the beets in quarters, and whirl them in a blender or food processor with a little of the beet liquid. Pour the processed beets and their liquid into a large glass pitcher. Add the lemon juice, honey, and Vege-Sal. Process the yogurt with 1 cup of the beet mixture in a blender or food processor until the ingredients are smooth. Pour the yogurt into the pitcher, whisk the ingredients well, adjust the seasonings, chill the soup, and serve it.

Yield: 8 bowl portions or 16 punch cups.

TOFU-SPINACH SOUP

Using fryers or broilers for making broth does not result in as rich and flavorful a product as broth made with a roaster.

CHICKEN BROTH

Neck, wings, and back of a roasting chicken (reserve the legs and breasts for another use)
8 cups water
1 teaspoon Vege-Sal
1 pound fresh spinach, washed, with stems removed
½ pound tofu, finely diced

To make the chicken broth, put the chicken neck, wings, and back in a soup pot with the water. Cover the pot, and simmer the broth all day. Strain the broth, discarding the solids. Pour the broth into a bowl, and set the bowl in the refrigerator overnight. Skim the fat off the top of the broth. This will yield about 6 cups of broth.

In a saucepan, bring the broth to a boil. Add the Vege-Sal and spinach. When the broth returns to a boil, turn off the heat, and add the tofu. Allow the tofu to heat through—about 5 to 8 minutes. Serve the soup immediately.

Yield: 4 servings.

VEGETABLE SOUP

8 cups water
2 tablespoons split peas
1 tablespoon barley
1 small potato, scrubbed and diced
2 stalks celery, diced
1 large onion, peeled and diced
3 medium carrots, scrubbed and sliced
1 turnip, rutabaga, *or* any other root vegetable, peeled and diced (optional)
6–8 fresh string beans, 1 cup peas, *or* another green vegetable
Vege-Sal, to taste
Dried basil, to taste

Bring the water to a boil in a soup pot. Add the split peas, barley, potato, celery, onion, carrots, and the root vegetable to the pot, and simmer the soup until the barley is tender—about 30 minutes. Ten minutes before serving, add the green vegetable, Vege-Sal, and basil, and cook the soup until the vegetable is tender.

Yield: 6 servings.

Main Dishes (Poultry, Fish, Meat, Vegetarian)

BROWN RICE AND CHICKEN

1 cup raw brown rice, rinsed

4 tablespoons unrefined sesame oil

3 cups chicken broth

2 onions, peeled and chopped

2 tablespoons sweet butter

2 stalks celery, chopped

2 cups cooked chicken, diced

1 tablespoon dry white wine

2 tablespoons unblanched almonds, finely ground

In a saucepan, sauté the rice in the sesame oil until all grains of rice are coated with the oil. Add the broth, bring the broth to a boil, reduce the heat, cover the pan, and simmer the liquid until the rice is almost tender—about 40 minutes.

In a frying pan, brown the onions in butter, add the celery, and cook the mixture until the vegetables are tender. Combine the vegetables with the rice mixture. Add the chicken, wine, and ground almonds, and cook the mixture 5 minutes longer. Serve the dish immediately.

Yield: 4 servings.

ROAST-CHICKEN CASSEROLE

1 5–6-pound roasting chicken (reserve the liver)
2 tablespoons garlic powder
2 tablespoons sweet paprika
½ pound fresh mushrooms, sliced
2 onions, peeled and minced

3 slices whole-wheat bread, crumbled
1 teaspoon poultry seasoning *or* stuffing herbs
Vege-Sal, to taste
1 tablespoon dried basil
1 tablespoon marjoram

Preheat the oven to 325°.

Wash and dry the chicken, removing as much fat as possible. Place the chicken in a roasting pan, and sprinkle the bird with the garlic powder and paprika. Bake the chicken for 1 hour. (Take care not to overcook the chicken—the meat should be juicy, not dry.) Set aside the pan with its drippings. When the chicken is cool enough to handle, remove the meat from the carcass, cutting it up into bite-sized pieces.

Wash and cut up the chicken liver. Cook it in the reserved drippings in the roasting pan. Add the mushrooms and onions to the pan, and cook them slightly—either in the oven or on top of the stove. Add the crumbled bread, poultry seasoning or stuffing herbs, Vege-Sal, basil, and marjoram. Return the chicken pieces to the roasting pan, mixing them well with the other ingredients. Put the mixture into a casserole, cover it, and place it in the oven on the lowest heat (150°) until it is time to serve.

Yield: 8 to 10 servings.

OPEN DEEP-DISH CHICKEN PIE

WHEAT-GERM PIE CRUST

1 cup wheat germ
½ cup (1 stick) sweet butter
½ teaspoon Vege-Sal

FILLING

4 cups roasted chicken meat, diced and seasoned with Vege-Sal, freshly ground pepper, and poultry seasoning
3 eggs, lightly beaten
1 cup dry white wine
1 cup chicken broth
2 cups fresh peas, cooked
4 hard-boiled eggs, coarsely chopped

½ cup toasted wheat germ

Preheat the oven to 350°.

To make the pie crust, blend thoroughly all the crust ingredients. Turn the mixture into an oiled deep-dish pie plate, pressing the crust firmly to the plate's sides and bottom. Bake the crust for 8 minutes, remove it from the oven, and cool it completely before filling it.

Turn the oven up to 375°.

Make the filling by combining all the filling ingredients. Turn the filling into the cooled deep-dish pie crust. Bake the pie for about 10 minutes. Lower the oven temperature to 300°, and bake the pie for another 25 minutes. Remove the pie from the oven, and sprinkle the top of the pie with the toasted wheat germ.

Yield: 8 to 10 servings.

ROAST DUCK

Earlier, I wrote about a New Year's Eve dinner party at which I served roast duck with wild rice. Brown rice or kasha (see p. 101) would also be a good accompaniment. And cranberry sauce (see p. 104) could be substituted for the chutney (see p. 103).

1 4–5 pound duck, with as much fat as possible removed	1 tablespoon garlic powder
	Vege-Sal, to taste
1 tablespoon sweet paprika	1 tablespoon poultry seasoning

Preheat the oven to 400°.

Wash the duck, and dry it with a paper towel. Sprinkle the duck with the remaining ingredients, and place it in the oven on a rack in a roasting pan for 20 minutes. Without opening the oven door, turn down the heat to the lowest setting (150°), and continue roasting the duck for 3 hours. Pour off the rendered fat from the roasting pan, and roast the duck for another 3 hours.

Yield: 4 small servings.

POACHED SALMON

Suggested menu: beet soup (borscht); poached salmon; brown rice or wild rice or a combination of the two; string beans, cauliflower, and sweet red peppers; cabbage salad; pound cake; watermelon, cherry, and blueberry dessert.

COURT BOUILLON

4 cups water
1 small onion, peeled and stuck with 2 cloves
1 slice lemon
4 peppercorns
½ bay leaf
Top half of 1 leafy stalk celery
2 sprigs parsley
1½ teaspoons Vege-Sal

1 6–8-pound salmon
Parsley for garnish
Lemon slices for garnish

To make the poaching liquid, place all the court-bouillon ingredients in a large fish poacher. Bring the liquid to a boil, reduce the heat, cover the poacher, and simmer the bouillon for 15 minutes.

Wash the salmon, place it on the rack in the fish poacher, cover the poacher, and simmer the fish for 20 minutes. Allow the fish to sit in the bouillon for a few minutes after the heat has been turned off. Transfer the salmon to a large serving platter, and garnish the fish with parsley and lemon slices.

Yield: at least 12 servings.

SALMON SOUFFLÉ WITH TOMATO SAUCE

TOMATO SAUCE

2–3 fresh tomatoes, diced
1 large onion, peeled and minced
1 tablespoon sweet butter
2–3 leaves fresh basil, minced, *or* 1 teaspoon dried basil
1 teaspoon Vege-Sal

SALMON SOUFFLÉ

4 cups fresh steamed salmon, cut into small pieces
2 eggs, beaten
2 cups milk
2 slices whole-wheat bread, crumbled
Vege-Sal, to taste
Garlic powder, to taste
Sweet paprika, to taste

To make the sauce, place the tomatoes, onion, butter, basil, and Vege-Sal in a small saucepan over low heat. Cover the pan. Do no add water—the tomatoes and onions will cook in their own juices. Cook the sauce for 12 minutes.

While the sauce is cooking, preheat the oven to 350°. Place the salmon in a soufflé dish. Combine the eggs, milk, bread, Vege-Sal, and garlic powder. Mix these with the salmon, and sprinkle the top of the mixture with the paprika. Bake the soufflé for about 40 minutes or until it is fairly firm. Serve it with the tomato sauce.

Yield: 5 to 6 servings.

BAKED TROUT WITH TOFU

3 fresh tomatoes,
    chopped
1 onion, peeled and
    chopped
2 medium-sized fresh
    trout (¾ pound
    each after scaling,
    gutting, and
    removal of head
    and fins)

Unrefined sesame oil
½ pound tofu, drained
    and cut into small
    cubes

Preheat the oven to 350°.

Place the tomatoes and onion in a roasting pan. Rinse the fish, and dry them with a paper towel. Rub the fish with some sesame oil, and place them in the roasting pan on top of the vegetables. Bake the fish for about 30 minutes or until the skin loosens and pulls away from the flesh. Put the tofu in the pan with the fish, close the oven door, and, with the oven turned off, allow the tofu to sit in the oven for about 10 minutes. Stir the tofu gently in the pan juices, and serve the dish immediately.

Yield: 4 servings.

LEG OF LAMB

Suggested menu: beet soup (borscht); leg of lamb; scalloped potatoes; string beans, cauliflower, and sweet red peppers; cabbage salad; mango chutney; stewed peaches or plums in honey.

1 5–7 pound leg of lamb	1 tablespoon dried basil
1 tablespoon sweet paprika	1 tablespoon dried marjoram
1 tablespoon garlic powder	

Preheat the oven to 400°.

Place the lamb in a roasting pan, and generously sprinkle the meat with the remaining ingredients. Cover the roasting pan. Roast the lamb for 20 minutes, reduce the heat to 150°, and roast the lamb for 6 hours more. The meat will be pink, tender, and juicy.

Yield: at least 7 servings, with leftovers.

LAMB STEW

Once in a while, I put up this stew while we play tennis. By the time we finish, the stew is done. I serve a green vegetable and guacamole with it, plus some corn on the cob.

3–4 shoulder lamb
chops
½ cup split peas
½ cup adzuki beans
1 large onion, peeled
and chopped
1 tomato, chopped

1–2 carrots, scrubbed
and sliced
Vege-Sal, to taste
3 tablespoons good dry
red wine

Wash the chops, and pat them dry with a paper towel.
Cube the meat, leaving the bones in. Brown the lamb
in a skillet (it is not necessary to add butter or oil),
and set the skillet aside. Combine the split peas, adzuki beans, onion, tomato, carrots, and Vege-Sal in
a pot with a cover and a heavy bottom, and add the
browned lamb. Pour the wine in the skillet in which
you have cooked the lamb, and stir the wine to loosen
the brown bits sticking to the pan. Add this to the
stew pot, cover the pot, and cook the stew over low
heat for 2 hours or until the meat and beans are tender.

Yield: 4 generous servings.

MEAT LOAF

1 pound ground lean
beef
1 onion, peeled and
minced
2 eggs, beaten
½ teaspoon Vege-Sal
1 fresh tomato,
chopped
1 clove garlic, peeled
and minced

1 teaspoon sweet
paprika
2–3 fresh basil leaves,
minced
½ cup milk
½ teaspoon freshly
ground black
pepper
2 slices whole-wheat
bread, crumbled

Preheat the oven to 325°.

Combine all the ingredients in a baking dish. Bake the meat loaf for about 40 minutes or until it is firm.

Yield: 6 servings.

EGGPLANT PARMIGIANA

1 large eggplant,
washed and thinly
sliced
4 fresh tomatoes,
finely chopped

1 pound whole-milk
mozzarella, thinly
sliced
Vege-Sal, to taste

Preheat the oven to 400°.

In a buttered baking dish, place alternating layers of eggplant, tomatoes, and mozzarella, sprinkling each layer with Vege-Sal and making sure to end with a layer of cheese. Bake the dish for 45 minutes.

Yield: 6 servings.

BROWN-RICE AND
CHEDDAR CASSEROLE

1 onion, peeled and
    chopped
2 stalks celery,
    chopped
1/2 pound mushrooms,
    sliced
1 clove garlic, peeled
    and minced
2 tablespoons sweet
    butter
1 teaspoon sweet
    paprika

1/2 teaspoon ginger
Vege-Sal, to taste
1/2 cup chopped
    parsley
3 cups cooked brown
    rice
1 pound Cheddar,
    grated or cut into
    small cubes

Preheat the oven to 350°.

In a large frying pan, lightly sauté the onion, celery, mushrooms, and garlic in the butter. Season the mixture with the paprika, ginger, and Vege-Sal, and stir in the parsley. Add the rice and cheese, and combine the ingredients well. Transfer the mixture to a baking dish, and bake the casserole for 30 minutes. Serve it hot.

Yield: 6 or more servings.

BROWN-RICE AND LEEK CASSEROLE

Norman can eat brown rice three times a day, so I make it quite often. Sometimes, for variety, I add a cupful of wheat berries to the pot, thereby providing a little crunch and a great deal of extra nutrition.

4–5 leeks
3 tablespoons
    unrefined olive oil
2 tablespoons sweet
    butter
1 teaspoon Vege-Sal
½ teaspoon sweet
    paprika

½ teaspoon garlic
    powder
1 cup raw brown rice
2 fresh tomatoes,
    chopped
1½ cups hot lamb
    stock *or* chicken
    stock

Preheat the oven to 325°.

Slice the leeks in half lengthwise, and wash them carefully. Chop them, and, in a 2-quart casserole, cook them in the oil and butter until they are tender but not browned. Stir in the Vege-Sal, paprika, garlic powder, rice, tomatoes, and stock, and bring the mixture to a boil. Cover the casserole, and bake it for 30 minutes or until all the liquid is absorbed and the rice is tender but not sticky.

Yield: 6 servings.

COUSCOUS

Millet has more protein than rice, corn, or oats and is higher in the amino acid lysine than other cereal grains. It is also a good source of B vitamins, phosphorous, iron, manganese, and copper.

2 cups uncooked whole
    millet *or* raw
    brown rice
4 cups water
1 teaspoon Vege-Sal
2 tablespoons sweet
    butter
1 large onion, peeled
    and diced
2–3 stalks celery, cut
    lengthwise and
    thinly sliced

4 medium-sized
    carrots, scrubbed
    and sliced
2 small zucchinis,
    quartered
    lengthwise and
    sliced
2–3 fresh tomatoes,
    chopped
1 large sweet red
    pepper, chopped
Diced cooked chicken
    or lamb (optional)

In a large covered saucepan, simmer the millet or rice in the water with the Vege-Sal and 1 tablespoon of the butter for 25 to 30 minutes or until the grain is tender.

Meanwhile, in a separate covered pot over low heat, cook the onion, celery, carrots, zucchinis, tomatoes, and pepper in the remaining tablespoon of butter until the carrots are tender but not soft. Do not add water. Cooked chicken or lamb may also be added.

Serve the vegetables on top of the hot millet or rice.

Yield: 4 to 5 servings.

CHEESE PIT

From a recipe given to me by Maxine Gomberg.

Not infrequently, I find myself with a number of people at the house at noon, and it becomes obvious that they will need to be fed. For example, not long ago, a television crew was taping Norman; the session took longer than expected. "There are only six of them," Norman said. "What can you do?" On such occasions, I can usually conjure up a pretty good fast meal, if I have the makings for a large cheese pit and a cabbage salad.

4 cups milk
6 eggs
1 teaspoon dried mustard
1 teaspoon sweet paprika
1–2 pinches cayenne
1 teaspoon garlic powder

Vege-Sal, to taste
6 slices whole-wheat bread, cubed or crumbled
1 pound sharp Cheddar, cubed
Paprika for topping

Preheat the oven to 375°.

Combine the milk, eggs, mustard, paprika, cayenne, garlic powder, and Vege-Sal in a blender. Put the bread in a large oven-proof dish, and pour this mixture over the bread. Add the cheese, and stir the ingredients until they are well mixed. Sprinkle the top of the cheese pit with paprika. Place the dish in the oven, and bake the cheese pit until its middle is firm. Serve the cheese pit immediately.

Yield: 8 to 10 servings.

Side Dishes and Condiments

LENTILS IN TOMATO SAUCE

1 onion, peeled and
    diced
1 tablespoon sweet
    butter
1 fresh tomato,
    chopped
1 sweet red pepper,
    cored, seeded, and
    diced

1 cup lentils, cooked
    until tender
Vege-Sal, to taste

In a saucepan, brown the onion slightly in the butter.
Add the tomato, and cook the vegetables for about 10
minutes. Add to the tomato-onion mixture the sweet
pepper, cooked lentils, and Vege-Sal. Stir the mixture
over low heat until it is heated through.

Yield: 4 servings.

LENTIL AND MILLET CAKES WITH TOMATO SAUCE

TOMATO SAUCE

1 onion, peeled and
  diced
1–2 fresh tomatoes,
  chopped
Vege-Sal, to taste

LENTIL AND MILLET
  CAKES

1 cup dried lentils,
  washed
¾ cup millet
2–3 cups vegetable
  broth, chicken
  broth, *or* water

1 onion, peeled and
  chopped
1 tablespoon sweet
  butter, plus
  additional butter
  for frying
2 eggs, beaten
2 tablespoons wheat
  germ
Vege-Sal, to taste
Freshly ground
  pepper, to taste

Make the tomato sauce by cooking the onion and tomatoes in a small covered saucepan over low heat for
15 to 20 minutes. Do not add water. Season the sauce
with the Vege-Sal.

To make the lentil and millet cakes, cook the lentils
and millet in separate saucepans in the broth or water
until the grains are done—about 30 minutes. Meanwhile, in a frying pan, cook the onion in the butter.
Combine well the lentils, millet, onion, eggs, wheat
germ, Vege-Sal, and pepper in a mixing bowl. Form
the mixture into cakes. Using the same frying pan in
which the onion was cooked, add more butter to the
pan, and fry the cakes until they are brown on both
sides. Serve the cakes hot with the tomato sauce.

Yield: 8 servings.

SESAME RICE

2 cups brown rice	3–4 tablespoons
4 cups boiling water	toasted sesame
1 teaspoon Vege-Sal	seeds (see Note on
	p. 70)

Add the rice to the boiling water. Cover the pot, and reduce the heat to low. Cook the rice until it is tender and all the water has been absorbed—about 40 minutes. Add the Vege-Sal. Serve the rice sprinkled with the sesame seeds.

Yield: 4 to 6 servings.

KASHA

Kasha is one of the best accompaniments to roast beef or leg of lamb. Serve this with side dishes of beets and red onion with vinaigrette, a green vegetable, and cabbage salad, and you've got a wonderful meal.

2 cups whole-grain buckwheat groats (kasha)	1 onion, peeled and minced
2 eggs, beaten	6–8 mushrooms, sliced
2 tablespoons sweet butter	Vege-Sal, to taste
	4 cups boiling chicken broth *or* water

Place the groats in a large unheated skillet. Add the eggs, and stir the mixture until all of the groats are covered with egg. Turn the heat on low, and continue stirring the groats until each grain is separate and slightly toasted—about 12 minutes. Remove the kasha from the heat, and set it aside.

Melt the butter in a casserole. Add the onion and brown it slightly; then add the mushrooms, and continue cooking the mixture for 1 to 2 minutes. Add the reserved kasha and the Vege-Sal, and mix the ingredients well. Pour the boiling broth or water into the groats, cover the casserole, and place the dish over low heat. Cook the kasha for about 40 minutes or until the broth or water is completely absorbed and each grain is fluffy and tender.

Yield: 6 to 8 generous servings.

RED BEANS MEXICAN STYLE

5 cups water	1 tablespoon sweet
2 cups dried red	butter
beans, rinsed and	2 fresh tomatoes,
picked over	chopped
1 onion, peeled and	¼ cup blackstrap
thinly sliced	molasses (I use
2 tablespoons	Plantation
unrefined sesame	brand)
oil *or* olive oil	1½ teaspoons Vege-Sal
	1 teaspoon dry
	mustard
	1 teaspoon chili
	powder

In a pot over high heat, bring the water to a boil, and add the beans slowly to the water. Reduce the heat, and cover the pot. Cook the beans for about 2 hours or until they are tender.

Meanwhile, in a skillet, cook the onion in the oil and butter for 15 minutes or until the onion is tender.

Add the tomatoes, and simmer the mixture until the tomatoes are thoroughly cooked—about 15 minutes.

When the beans are done, combine them with the onion-tomato mixture, molasses, Vege-Sal, mustard, and chili powder. Cook the mixture over low heat for at least 15 minutes. Serve the dish hot.

Yield: 6 to 8 servings.

MANGO CHUTNEY

Whenever I serve lamb, beef, or poultry to guests, I offer this chutney. If you do the same, be prepared to supply your friends with the recipe. The chutney will last for at least a month in the refrigerator.

3 ripe mangoes, peeled
    and cubed
2 cloves garlic, peeled
    and crushed or
    minced
1 onion, peeled and
    chopped
Juice of 2 limes *or*
    lemons
4 tablespoons honey,
    or to taste
1 whole lemon,
    chopped
Peel of 1 orange,
    minced
3 cups raisins

½ fresh pineapple,
    peeled, cored,
    and diced
12 kumquats, chopped
    (optional)
1 teaspoon nutmeg
1 teaspoon cinnamon
1 teaspoon ginger
6 cloves, crushed
1 teaspoon Vege-Sal
1 teaspoon freshly
    ground pepper

Combine the mangoes, garlic, onion, lime or lemon juice, and honey in a large saucepan, and simmer the mixture for 10 minutes. Add the other ingredients, and simmer the chutney for another 20 minutes. Put the chutney in clean jars, and store it in the refrigerator.

Yield: 4 cups.

CRANBERRY SAUCE

1 12-ounce package fresh cranberries, washed, stemmed, and picked over	2–3 tablespoons honey or to taste

Put the berries in a large pot, add the honey, cover the pot, and bring the fruit to a boil. Watch the pot carefully so that it doesn't boil over. Turn off the heat, and let the pot sit on the hot burner until the berries stop cooking.

Yield: about 2 cups.

Vegetables

POTATO PANCAKES

5–6 potatoes (about 2
    pounds),
    unpeeled,
    scrubbed, and cut
    into small pieces
3 eggs, beaten
3 tablespoons whole-
    wheat flour

1 large onion, peeled
    and minced
Vege-Sal, to taste
Butter (for greasing
    the griddle)

Grind the potatoes in a blender or food processor. Combine the potatoes with the eggs, flour, onion, and Vege-Sal. Drop 1 large tablespoonful of the mixture for each pancake onto a hot buttered griddle. Brown the pancakes on both sides, and serve them hot.

Yield: about 15 pancakes.

SCALLOPED POTATOES

2 cups sliced raw
    unpeeled
    potatoes
1½ tablespoons whole-
    wheat flour
Vege-Sal, to taste
1 onion, peeled and
    finely diced

1½ cups grated sharp
    Cheddar
2 tablespoons sweet
    butter
3 cups milk
    (approximately)

Preheat the oven to 300°.

Put a layer of potatoes in the bottom of a baking dish, sprinkling the potatoes with some flour and some Vege-Sal. Then put down a layer of onions and a layer of Cheddar. Continue the layering process (ending with the Cheddar) until the potatoes, onion, and cheese have been used up. Dot the top layer with small pieces of the butter. Add enough milk almost to cover the top layer. Cover the dish, and bake the potatoes for about 30 minutes or until they are tender.

Yield: 3 to 4 servings.

OVEN-BAKED POTATO WEDGES

Combining white potatoes with sweet potatoes enhances the flavor of both. This dish is a good accompaniment to any kind of meat.

1 tablespoon sweet
   butter
1 tablespoon unrefined
   sesame oil
3 sweet potatoes,
   unpeeled and
   quartered

3 white potatoes,
   unpeeled and
   quartered
1 large onion, peeled
   and sliced
Vege-Sal, to taste
Sweet paprika, to taste

Preheat the oven to 350°.

Melt the butter in baking dish, and add the oil. Turn the potatoes in the butter and oil until all the pieces are well coated. Add the onion, and sprinkle the dish with Vege-Sal and paprika. Bake the wedges for 30 to 40 minutes or until the potatoes are golden brown and fork-tender.

Yield: about 8 servings.

RED, WHITE, AND GREEN

An attractive and delicious three-vegetable dish for festive occasions.

2 pounds string beans,
   washed and cut on
   an angle into 1½-
   inch pieces
1 head cauliflower,
   broken into small
   flowerets
2 sweet red bell
   peppers, seeded
   and cut in narrow
   strips about 2
   inches long

1 tablespoon sweet
   butter
1 tablespoon unrefined
   olive oil
Vege-Sal, to taste

Cook the string beans and cauliflower in a little water in separate covered pots. Do not overcook the vegetables—the string beans take longer to cook (about 10 minutes) than the cauliflower (about 5 minutes). You want the beans to be tender and bright green, and the cauliflower fairly crisp.

In a frying pan, sauté the peppers briefly in the butter. Do not allow the peppers to get limp. Remove the peppers from the heat, and add the olive oil.

Just before serving, combine the vegetables, tossing them gently with the Vege-Sal and any oil left in the pan in which the peppers were sautéed. Serve the vegetables on a warm platter.

Yield: 15 servings.

ZUCCHINI

2 small zucchinis,
    quartered
    lengthwise and
    sliced
1 large onion, peeled
    and diced

2 fresh tomatoes,
    chopped
1 tablespoon sweet
    butter

Combine all the ingredients, and place them in a covered pot over very low heat. Do not add water—the vegetables will cook in their own juices. And be sure not to overcook the vegetables—6 to 8 minutes should be long enough.

Yield: about 4 servings.

CELERY ROOT

For a pleasant and unusual taste, celery root deserves to be served more often.

1 large celery root, peeled and julienned or grated	1½–2 tablespoons sweet butter Vege-Sal, to taste

In a frying pan, quickly cook the celery root in the butter, stirring constantly. Do not overcook the vegetable. Add the Vege-Sal, and serve the celery root immediately.

Yield: about 4 servings.

EGGPLANT AND TOMATO

1 eggplant, unpeeled and diced	5–6 fresh basil leaves, chopped, *or* 1 tablespoon dried basil
2 fresh tomatoes, chopped	
1 onion, peeled and chopped	1 tablespoon sweet butter
4–5 mushrooms, sliced	Vege-Sal, to taste

Combine all the ingredients in a saucepan. Cover the pan, and cook the vegetables over low heat for about 6 to 8 minutes. Do not add liquid—the vegetables will cook in their own juices.

Yield: 3 to 4 servings.

ACORN-SQUASH PUFF

2 tablespoons sweet
    butter
    (approximately)
3 1/2-pound acorn
    squash, washed,
    cut in half
    widthwise, and
    seeded
1/2 cup blackstrap
    molasses
3 tablespoons whole-
    wheat flour

1 teaspoon Vege-Sal
1/4 teaspoon nutmeg
1/4 teaspoon ginger
3 eggs, separated
1/2 cup finely chopped
    pecans or walnuts

Preheat the oven to 400°.

Place a small piece of butter (about 1 teaspoon) in each squash half, and bake the squash until they are done. Keep the oven on.

Scoop out the squash meat from the shell, and, in a mixing bowl, combine the squash with the molasses, flour, Vege-Sal, nutmeg, ginger, and egg yolks. Beat the egg whites until they are stiff but not dry. Gently fold the whites into the squash mixture. Turn the squash into a buttered baking dish, sprinkle the chopped nuts over the top, and bake the puff for 45 minutes or until the top is golden and crusty.

Yield: 6 servings.

Breads

PECAN LOAF

2 cups raw, unsalted
  pecans, chopped
1 onion, peeled and
  chopped
1 cup chopped fresh
  tomatoes
1 cup whole-wheat
  bread crumbs
2 eggs, beaten

½ cup milk
Vege-Sal, to taste
Freshly ground
  pepper, to taste
½ teaspoon sage
1 tablespoon melted
  butter

Preheat the oven to 350°.

Combine the pecans, onion, tomatoes, bread crumbs, eggs, milk, Vege-Sal, pepper, and sage. Place the mixture in a 9×5×3-inch buttered loaf pan, and brush the top of the loaf with the melted butter. Bake the pecan loaf for 35 minutes. Serve it while it is hot.

Yield: 1 loaf.

WHOLE-WHEAT BREAD

2 packages dry yeast
1/2 cup lukewarm
    (between 105°
    and 115°) water
1/2 teaspoon honey
2 cups milk
1 cup (2 sticks) butter
    plus extra for
    greasing the bowl
    and the bread
    pans

1/2 cup honey
7 1/2 cups stone-ground
    whole-wheat
    flour
3 eggs, beaten
1 tablespoon salt
1/2 cup stone-ground
    corn meal
    (optional)

Proof the yeast by dissolving it in the water. Add the 1/2 teaspoon of honey. Mix the ingredients well, and set the mixture aside until it bubbles.

Warm the milk in a small saucepan over low heat, and melt the butter in the milk. Stir in the 1/2 cup of honey. In a large mixing bowl, combine 3 cups of the flour with the eggs and the milk-butter-honey mixture. Add the proofed yeast to the flour mixture when the latter has cooled to lukewarm. Beat the mixture well. Set it in a warm place for 15 minutes.

Add the salt, the optional corn meal, and the remaining 4 1/2 cups of flour. Turn the dough out onto a floured surface, and knead the dough for 10 minutes. Scrape the mixing bowl thoroughly, but do not wash it. Butter the bowl. Place the dough into the buttered bowl, and cover the dough with a clean cloth. Allow the dough to rise in a warm place until it has doubled in bulk—about 30 minutes.

Remove the dough from the bowl, knead it again for 10 minutes, divide it in thirds, and form each piece of dough into a loaf. Place each loaf in a buttered

9×5×3-inch bread pan, cover the pans with a clean cloth, and allow the dough to rise again for about 30 minutes or until it has doubled in bulk.

Preheat the oven to 350°.

Bake the breads for 45 minutes or until they are golden brown. Remove the loaves from the pan, and set them on a rack to cool.

Yield: 3 loaves.

CORN BREAD

When I entertain a large group—say, twenty people—I double this recipe, and bake it for 1 hour in a 16×10×2½-inch pan.

1 cup stone-ground corn meal
½ cup whole-wheat flour
1 tablespoon blackstrap molasses
½ teaspoon Vege-Sal
2 eggs, beaten
1 cup milk
1 onion, peeled and diced

2 sweet jalapeños, stemmed, seeded, and chopped
½ cup unrefined sesame oil
Fresh corn kernels cut from 3 ears of corn
½ pound sharp Cheddar, grated or diced
2 packages dry yeast

Combine all the ingredients, and pour the batter into a buttered 8×8-inch pan. Set the bread in a warm place for about 30 minutes to rise.

Preheat the oven to 375°.

Bake the bread for 40 minutes or until it is brown and crisp on top. Cut it into squares. Serve it hot.

Yield: 10 servings.

WHOLE-WHEAT BANANA BREAD

½ cup (1 stick) sweet butter
1 cup honey
2 eggs
2 cups whole-wheat flour
1 teaspoon Vege-Sal

1 package dry yeast
2 large ripe bananas, peeled and mashed
¼ cup plain yogurt

Preheat the oven to 350°.

In a large bowl, cream the butter and honey until the mixture is light and fluffy. Beat in the eggs. In another bowl, combine the flour, Vege-Sal, and yeast. In a third bowl, stir the bananas into the yogurt. Alternately add the flour mixture and banana mixture to the butter mixture, stirring just enough to combine the ingredients.

Turn the batter into a buttered 9×5-inch loaf pan. Bake the bread for 50 to 60 minutes or until the loaf is done. Cool the bread in the pan for 10 minutes. Remove the bread from the pan, and place it on a rack to finish cooling.

Yield: 1 loaf.

BRAN MUFFINS

1 package dry yeast	1 teaspoon Vege-Sal
1/2 cup warm (between 105° and 115°) water	3 eggs, beaten
	1/4 cup (1/2 stick) sweet butter, melted
1/2 teaspoon honey *or* maple syrup	1/2 cup honey *or* maple syrup
2 cups stone-ground whole-wheat flour	2 cups raisins
1/2 cup corn meal	Grated rind of 1 orange
1/2 cup wheat germ	Juice of 1 orange

Dissolve the yeast in the water, to which 1/2 teaspoon of honey or maple syrup has been added. Set the mixture aside. Combine the flour, corn meal, wheat germ, and Vege-Sal; then add the eggs, butter, the 1/2 cup of honey or maple syrup, the raisins, orange rind, and orange juice. Stir the mixture, and add the proofed yeast. Combine the ingredients well. Spoon the batter into buttered muffin tins, and set the batter in a warm place to rise for about 15 minutes.

Preheat the oven to 350°.

Bake the muffins for 30 minutes or until they are golden brown.

Yield: 12 muffins.

OATMEAL-BANANA MUFFINS

1 cup oatmeal flakes	½ cup honey
1 cup whole-wheat flour	½ cup sweet butter, melted
1 teaspoon Vege-Sal	1 ripe banana, peeled and mashed
2 eggs, separated	
½ cup milk, scalded	1 package dry yeast
1 teaspoon vanilla	

Preheat the oven to 375°.

Combine the oatmeal flakes, flour, and Vege-Sal in a mixing bowl. In another bowl, stir the egg yolks slightly, and add the hot milk; then beat the mixture until it becomes light and thick. Add the vanilla, honey, melted butter, and banana. Gently fold into this mixture the dry ingredients and the yeast. Set the bowl aside in a warm place for about 12 minutes.

Beat the egg whites until they are stiff but not dry, and fold them into the batter. Spoon the batter into buttered muffin tins until they are two-thirds full. Bake the muffins for 30 minutes or until they are golden brown. Remove the muffins from the tins, and cool them on a rack.

Yield: about 18 muffins.

ZUCCHINI OR CARROT BREAD

3 eggs
1 cup unrefined
    sesame oil
1½ cups honey
2 cups grated zucchini
    or carrots
2 teaspoons vanilla
2 cups whole-wheat
    flour

1 package dry yeast
1 tablespoon cinnamon
½ teaspoon nutmeg
1 teaspoon Vege-Sal
1 cup raisins
1 cup chopped walnuts

Beat the eggs slightly in a large mixing bowl. Add the oil, honey, zucchini or carrots, vanilla, flour, yeast, cinnamon, nutmeg, and Vege-Sal. Beat the ingredients until they are thoroughly blended. Stir in the raisins and walnuts. Spoon the batter into two buttered 9×5×3-inch loaf pans. Set the breads in a warm place to rise for 30 minutes.

Preheat the oven to 375°.

Bake the loaves for 1 hour. Remove the breads from the pans, and cool the loaves on a rack.

Yield: 2 loaves.

Salads

CHICKPEA SALAD

1 cup dried chickpeas,
    cooked until
    tender
1 small red onion,
    peeled and diced
8 sprigs parsley,
    chopped
1/4 cup unrefined
    sesame oil

Juice of 1 lemon
1/2 teaspoon Vege-Sal
1/4 teaspoon dry
    mustard
Freshly ground black
    pepper, to taste

In a bowl, combine the chickpeas, onions, and parsley. In a blender, blend the oil, lemon juice, Vege-Sal, mustard, and pepper, and pour this dressing over the chickpea mixture. Toss the salad lightly, and refrigerate it for at least 1 hour before serving.

Yield: about 4 servings.

CABBAGE SALAD

I serve this salad as a first course almost every night. There's a good reason for including each of its ingredients. *Cabbage:* Research at Johns Hopkins School of Hygiene and Public Health has shown that cabbage, Brussels sprouts, and broccoli contain chemicals that protect against cancer. *Garlic and red onion:* The *Longevity Letter* (July 1986), a monthly review of biomedical research related to life extension, reports on studies conducted over the last ten years that indicate that fresh raw garlic reduces serum cholesterol and triglyceride levels, and increases HDL cholesterol. Clinical tests also suggest that dietary garlic lowers the risk of some types of cancer. *Onion* has somewhat the same effect in the body as raw garlic. *Sweet red pepper and parsley* supply large amounts of vitamins A and C. *Red-clover or alfalfa sprouts* contain many minerals and vitamins C and K. *Jícama* (pronounced ''hee′ka-mah'') is a native Mexican root vegetable that I was not familiar with until I came to Los Angeles. It is crisp like a water chestnut and resembles a large potato with a very tough skin. It is eaten peeled and raw or cooked, is a source of potassium and vitamin C, and adds a wonderful taste and texture to salads. *Lemon juice* provides vitamin C and bioflavonoids. *Unrefined sesame oil or olive oil* provides the body with the kind of material that it needs to manufacture good cholesterol (see p. 27). Those interested in adding nutrition and fiber to their meals should include this salad—or one similar to it—in their diet.

¼ (¾ pound) green
cabbage, cored
and finely sliced
1-2 cloves garlic,
peeled and
minced or
mashed
½ red onion, peeled
and finely minced
1 sweet red pepper,
seeded and
chopped

1 handful red-clover *or*
alfalfa sprouts
1 handful parsley
leaves, chopped
½ small jícama, peeled
and diced
Juice of 1 lemon,
unstrained
1-2 tablespoons
unrefined sesame
oil *or* olive oil

Combine all the ingredients. Chill the salad before serving.

Yield: about 8 servings.

FOUR-BEAN SALAD

I suppose most people would use canned beans when making this salad, but I would not. If I use a large pot for each kind of bean, it makes the job of cooking the beans much easier. Using twice as much water as beans, bring the water to a boil. Then turn the heat down, and cook the beans slowly for about 1 hour. Occasionally stir the beans, and check for doneness. Each kind of bean *must* be cooked separately.

1 cup peeled and
minced red onion
or minced
scallions, white
and green parts
1 clove garlic, peeled
and minced
½ teaspoon Vege-Sal
½ teaspoon dry
mustard
Juice of 1 lemon
3 tablespoons
unrefined olive oil

2 tablespoons minced
fresh parsley
1 cup cooked red
kidney beans
1 cup cooked white
beans (for
example,
cannellini or white
kidney)
1 cup cooked
chickpeas
1 cup cooked black
beans

To make the dressing, combine well the onion or
scallions, garlic, Vege-Sal, mustard, lemon juice, olive oil, and parsley in a bowl. Place the beans in a
salad bowl, and pour the dressing over them. Toss the
ingredients gently with a wooden spoon until the
beans are coated with the dressing. Serve the salad
chilled.

Yield: about 15 small servings.

TABBOULI

Every time I serve this salad, guests ask for the recipe. It is an extremely nourishing dish as well as a
tasty one.

2 cups raw cracked
    wheat
1 cup warm water
1 cup chopped parsley
1/2 cup peeled and
    chopped red
    onion
2 fresh tomatoes,
    chopped
1 large sweet red
    pepper, cored,
    seeded, and
    chopped
2 tablespoons fresh
    mint, minced
Juice of 1 lemon
1/2 cup unrefined
    sesame oil *or*
    olive oil
Vege-Sal, to taste
Freshly ground
    pepper, to taste

In a bowl, soak the cracked wheat in the water for 1 hour. Combine well the remaining ingredients in another bowl. Mix the soaked wheat into the vegetable mixture, place the tabbouli in the refrigerator, and allow the wheat to absorb the other flavors.

Yield: about 10 servings.

BEET AND RED-ONION VINAIGRETTE

1 bunch fresh beets,
    scrubbed
1–2 cups water
Juice of 1 lemon
2 teaspoons honey
2 tablespoons
    unrefined olive oil
Vege-Sal, to taste
1/2 red onion, peeled
    and finely minced

Cut the stems off of the beets, leaving about 1 1/2 inches, so that the beets will not lose their juice while cooking. Place the beets in a pressure cooker with 1 cup of water or in a regular covered pot with 2 cups of water, and cook the vegetable until it is tender (the pressure cooker will do the job in 15 minutes; the regular pot will take twice as long). Remove the beet skins with paper towels, and slice the beets. Combine the lemon juice, honey, oil and Vege-Sal in a bowl. Add the sliced beets and the onion to the dressing, mixing the ingredients well.

Yield: 3 to 4 servings.

Desserts

RICE PUDDING

4 cups cooked short-
    grain brown rice
3 eggs, beaten
3 cups milk
½ cup honey

½ teaspoon Vege-Sal
1 teaspoon vanilla
2 cups raisins
Cinnamon

Preheat the oven to 350°.

Combine the rice, eggs, milk, honey, Vege-Sal, vanilla, and raisins in a baking dish. Sprinkle the top of
the pudding with cinnamon. Bake the pudding for
about 30 minutes.

Yield: 5 to 6 servings.

CUSTARD

4 cups milk
6 eggs
½ teaspoon vanilla

3 tablespoons honey
Cinnamon

Preheat the oven to 350°.

Put about 1 cup of the milk in a blender; add the eggs, vanilla, and honey; and blend the ingredients. Combine this mixture with the remaining 3 cups of milk, and pour this into individual custard cups or one large bowl, if you prefer. Sprinkle the top of the custard with cinnamon. Place the cups or bowl in a shallow pan containing a few inches of water, put the pan in the oven, and bake the custard until it is set—about 40 minutes. Keep a close watch on the custard so that it doesn't overcook. Refrigerate the custard, and serve it plain or topped with fresh blueberries or any other raw or cooked berry or fruit.

Yield: 6 to 8 servings.

STRAWBERRY-BANANA-YOGURT DESSERT

Norman usually eats a banana a day. But sometimes they sit in the fruit bowl too long and turn brown. At this point, I peel them, place them in a covered dish, and freeze them. Then I have to think of some way to use them. Once, someone gave us four boxes of beautiful strawberries. Since Norman doesn't like fresh strawberries, I stewed them in some honey. Then I decided to combine the frozen bananas and the strawberries in the blender with some yogurt and to use it as a frozen dessert. Norman thought it was very good. Now I also give it to him as a cold drink on hot afternoons. When I don't have frozen bananas, I use fresh ones. Almost every time I make this recipe, I vary it slightly. But it's delicious no matter how you prepare it.

1 pint ripe sweet strawberries	Ripe bananas, peeled and fresh or frozen
2 tablespoons honey	1–2 cups plain yogurt

Stew the strawberries in the honey, and put them in the refrigerator. Cut the bananas in thirds, and place them, with a few tablespoons of the stewed strawberries and the yogurt in the blender, and combine the ingredients well. Serve this as a drink, or place the mixture in the freezer until it is slightly frozen and serve it as dessert.

Yield: 4 servings for every 3 bananas.

POUND CAKE

2 cups (4 sticks) sweet butter	½ teaspoon Vege-Sal
1½ cups honey	1 teaspoon vanilla
10 eggs, separated	Grated rind of 1 lemon *or* orange
4½ cups (1 pound) stone-ground whole-wheat flour	Juice of 1 lemon *or* orange

Preheat the oven to 300°.

Beat the butter and honey in a mixing bowl until the mixture is creamy and fluffy. Slowly add the egg yolks, and beat the mixture well. Gradually add the flour and Vege-Sal, and continue beating the mixture. Stir in the vanilla, lemon or orange rind, and lemon or orange juice.

In another bowl, whip the egg whites until they are stiff but not dry, and fold them into the batter.

Pour the batter into two buttered loaf pans, each 5×10×3 inches, and bake the cakes for 1 hour 30 minutes or until the cakes shrink from the sides of the pans and a cake tester inserted into the cakes comes out clean. Remove the cakes from the pans, cool them on a rack, and serve them with the watermelon, cherry, and blueberry dessert (below).

Yield: 2 loaves.

WATERMELON, CHERRY, AND BLUEBERRY DESSERT

1 medium-sized ripe, sweet watermelon (about 9 pounds)	3 pounds ripe sweet cherries
	1 pint fresh blueberries

Using a melon baller, scoop out the watermelon, avoiding the seeds. Wash the cherries, cut them in half, and remove the pits. Wash and pick over the blueberries. Combine the fruit in a large glass bowl, and refrigerate it until it is time to serve. The fruit may be served as is or with pound cake (above).

Yield: at least 15 servings.

CRANBERRY-APPLE CRISP

2 12-ounce packages
    fresh cranberries
    (about 4 cups),
    washed, picked
    over, and stems
    removed
6–8 apples (about 4
    pounds), peeled,
    cored, and sliced
1 ½ cups honey or to
    taste

1 ½ cups rolled oats
1 cup date sugar *or*
    honey, *or* maple
    syrup, to taste
1 teaspoon Vege-Sal
1 cup (2 sticks) sweet
    butter, cut into
    small pieces
1 pint heavy cream,
    whipped

Preheat the oven to 350°.

Combine the cranberries, apples, and honey in a large pot. Bring the mixture to a boil, turn off the heat, and allow the pot to sit on the burner while you prepare the rolled-oat mixture.

Combine well the rolled oats with the date sugar and Vege-Sal. Pour the cranberry-apple mixture into a 10×15×2-inch pan, spreading the mixture evenly. Sprinkle the rolled-oat mixture over the top, and place the small pieces of butter evenly over the oatmeal.

Bake the crisp for 1 hour. Cut it into squares, and put a dollop of whipped cream on each square.

Yield: about 10 servings.

APPLESAUCE

Whenever I stew any kind of fruit or berry, I use honey—only honey—no sugar, no water. You won't believe what a difference it makes until you try it.

The basic recipe is the same for all fruits and berries. (*Note:* Italian plums, halved and pitted, are especially good cooked this way.)

5–6 apples, peeled, cored, quartered, and sliced	**2–3 tablespoons honey or to taste**
½ cup raisins *or* 3–4 plums (optional)	

Put the apples in a large pot with the raisins or plums, if you wish. Add the honey, cover the pot, bring the fruit to a boil, turn the heat off immediately, and let the pot sit on the burner until the fruit has stopped cooking.

Yield: 4 to 5 servings.

STEWED PEARS

An excellent dessert to accompany a roast-duck entrée.

4 firm but ripe Bartlett pears, peeled but with the cores and stems intact	**2–3 tablespoons honey 3–4 cinnamon sticks**

Place the pears in a large saucepan. Add the honey and cinnamon sticks. Stew the pears over low heat, turning them over every 5 minutes or so, until they are cooked through. Test each pear for tenderness with a thin pointed knife. Chill the pears, and serve them in small glass bowls with some of the stewing liquid.

Yield: 4 servings.

CAROB BROWNIES

One of Norman's favorite dishes, which I make often. However, almost every time I make it, I change the recipe. Sometimes I use pecans instead of almonds, whole-wheat flour instead of wheat germ. This is the latest version and, I think, the best.

1 1/2 cups honey	3 eggs
1 cup (2 sticks) sweet butter	1/2 teaspoon vanilla
	1/2 teaspoon Vege-Sal
2 1/2 cups raw almonds, which have been pulverized in the blender	1 1/2 cups carob powder
	12 dates, pitted and diced (optional)
1 cup wheat germ	

Preheat the oven to 250°.

Combine the honey and butter in a saucepan over low heat, cover the pan, and melt the butter.

In a large bowl, mix together the almonds, wheat germ, eggs, vanilla, Vege-Sal, carob powder, and dates. Add the honey-butter mixture to the large bowl. Stir the ingredients well, pour the batter into a buttered 2 × 14 × 8-inch pan, and bake the brownies for about 1 hour or until a knife stuck in the middle of the brownies comes out clean. Cut the cake into small squares while it is still warm, and store the brownies in a covered tin in the refrigerator.

Yield: 12 brownies.

HAZELNUT TORTE

When I became interested in nutrition, I stopped buy-ing the white-flour- and sugar-laden birthday cakes our children had learned to expect whenever they had a birthday. Of course, I ran into a lot of opposition. But I won the battle by baking this cake and adorning it with lovely little wooden candle holders formed like winged angels. After that, no birthday was complete without those candle holders and this nut cake.

½ pound shelled raw
    hazelnuts
8 eggs, separated
1 cup honey
½ cup whole-wheat
    bread crumbs

Grated rind of 1 lemon
Juice of 1 lemon
1 teaspoon vanilla
1 cup raspberry jelly
    or strawberry jelly

Preheat the oven to 325°.

Grind the hazelnuts in a blender. Set aside 2 table-spoons of the ground nuts for decorating the cake.

In a bowl, beat the egg yolks with the honey until the mixture is light. Add the bread crumbs, lemon rind and juice, vanilla, and ground nuts. Beat the egg whites until they are stiff but not dry, and fold them into the batter. Pour the batter into two buttered 10-inch springform pans, and bake the layers for 30 min-utes. Cool the layers in the pans on a rack.

Remove the layers from the pans; spread the jelly between the layers, on top of the cake, and around the sides of the cake. Sprinkle the reserved ground hazelnuts on top of the torte.

Yield: 1 cake.

NUTRITIOUS NIBBLE

4 eggs, beaten
1 cup honey
1 cup chopped walnuts
1 cup unsweetened
 shredded coconut
1 cup chopped pitted
 dates
¾ cup whole-wheat
 flour

½ cup wheat germ
1 teaspoon blackstrap
 molasses
1 rounded tablespoon
 brewer's yeast
Cinnamon

Preheat the oven to 150°.

Combine all the ingredients except the cinnamon, and pour the batter into a buttered 9-inch square baking pan. Sprinkle the top with cinnamon. Bake the dessert for 20 minutes or until it is done. Cut the nibble into 1-inch squares.

Yield: 81 squares

OATMEAL COOKIES

These cookies come out moist and chewy if the dough is refrigerated overnight.

1 ½ cups oatmeal
   flakes
1 cup sweet-rice flour
½ cup wheat germ
1 cup (2 sticks) sweet
   butter, melted
1 cup maple syrup *or*
   honey

3 eggs
2 cups raisins
1 cup chopped walnuts
   or pecans
1 teaspoon Vege-Sal

Preheat the oven to 350°.

Combine the oatmeal flakes, sweet-rice flour, and wheat germ in a large bowl. Add the butter, maple syrup or honey, eggs, raisins, nuts, and Vege-Sal. Stir the ingredients well, and drop 1 tablespoonful of the dough for each cookie onto a buttered cookie sheet. Press the dough into the desired shape with the back of a spoon. Bake the cookies for about 6 minutes or until they are golden brown. Cool them on a rack.

Yield: 4 dozen cookies.

ALMOND MACAROON CAKE

Don't attempt to bake this cake in a very hot oven—the nut dough scorches easily. Bake it slowly, and keep an eye on it.

1½ cups honey
1 cup (2 sticks) sweet butter
1 pound (2½ cups) raw unblanched almonds, ground in the blender

5 tablespoons wheat germ
3 eggs, beaten
½ teaspoon almond extract
½ teaspoon Vege-Sal

Preheat the oven to 250°.

Place the honey and butter in a saucepan over low heat until the butter has melted.

In a large bowl, combine the almonds, wheat germ, eggs, almond extract, and Vege-Sal, and then add the honey-butter mixture. Stir the ingredients well. Transfer the batter to a buttered 2 × 14 × 8-inch pan. Bake the cake until a cake tester inserted into the middle of the cake comes out clean. While the cake is still warm, cut it into small squares. Store the squares in the refrigerator in a covered tin.

Yield: 12 squares.

Bibliography

Brody, Jane. *Jane Brody's Good Food Book.* New York: Norton, 1985.

Burkitt, Denis. *Western Diseases: Their Emergence and Prevention.* Cambridge, Mass.: Harvard University Press, 1969.

Clark, Linda. *The New Way to Eat.* Millbrae, Calif.: Celestial Arts, 1980.

Hunter, Beatrice Trim. *The Great Nutrition Robbery.* New York: Scribner's, 1978.

Painter, Neil S. *Diverticular Disease of the Colon: Deficiency Disease of Western Civilization.* London: Heineman, 1975.

Rohe, Fred. *The Complete Book of Natural Foods.* Boulder: Col.: Shambhala, 1983.

Shaeffer, John R., and Leonard A. Stevens. *Future Water.* New York: William Morrow, 1983.

Wurtman, Richard J., and Judith J. Wurtman, eds. *Nutrition and the Brain,* vol. 6. New York: Raven Press, 1983.

Index

Italicized page numbers refer
to recipes.

THE COMPLETE GUIDE TO A LIFETIME OF WELL-BEING BY AMERICA'S MOST TRUSTED HEALTH WRITER

JANE BRODY'S

The New York Times
— GUIDE TO —

PERSONAL HEALTH

Illustrated with graphs and charts, fully indexed and conveniently arranged under fifteen sections:

NUTRITION

EMOTIONAL HEALTH

ABUSED SUBSTANCES

EYES, EARS, NOSE AND
    THROAT

SAFETY

PESKY HEALTH PROBLEMS

COMMON KILLERS

EXERCISE

SEXUALITY AND
    REPRODUCTION

DENTAL HEALTH

ENVIRONMENTAL HEALTH
    EFFECTS

SYMPTOMS

COMMON SERIOUS
    ILLNESSES

MEDICAL CARE

COPING WITH HEALTH PROBLEMS

"Jane Brody's encyclopedia of wellness covers everything."
Washington Post

64121-6/$12.95 US/$16.75 Can